Elective Surgery - Challenges and Practice around the World

Edited by Marisa Domingues dos Santos and Donzília Sousa Silva

Published in London, United Kingdom

Elective Surgery - Challenges and Practice around the World
http://dx.doi.org/10.5772/intechopen.1003459
Edited by Marisa Domingues dos Santos and Donzília Sousa Silva

Contributors
Abel Mesquita, Ahmed Abdelbary, André Pinto, Aphrodite Fotiadou, Donzília Sousa Silva, Gil Levy,
Islam Ali Soliman ElSayed, Kyriacos Evangelou, Marisa D. Santos, Marisa Domingues dos Santos, Naama
Marcus, Nada Salama, Thalia Petropoulou, Waleed Mohamed Fadlalla, Zviya Fridman-Kogan

Notice

Statements and opinions expressed in the chapters are these of the individual contributors and not
necessarily those of the editors or publisher. No responsibility is accepted for the accuracy of
information contained in the published chapters. The publisher assumes no responsibility for any
damage or injury to persons or property arising out of the use of any materials, instructions, methods
or ideas contained in the book.

First published in London, United Kingdom, 2025 by IntechOpen
IntechOpen is the global imprint of INTECHOPEN LIMITED, registered in England and Wales,
registration number: 11086078, 167-169 Great Portland Street, London, W1W 5PF, United Kingdom

For EU product safety concerns: IN TECH d.o.o., Prolaz Marije Krucifikse Kozulić 3, 51000 Rijeka,
Croatia, info@intechopen.com or visit our website at intechopen.com.

British Library Cataloguing-in-Publication Data
A catalogue record for this book is available from the British Library

Elective Surgery - Challenges and Practice around the World
Edited by Marisa Domingues dos Santos and Donzília Sousa Silva
p. cm.
Print ISBN 978-1-83634-353-0
Online ISBN 978-1-83634-352-3
eBook (PDF) ISBN 978-1-83634-354-7

If disposing of this product, please recycle the paper responsibly.

IntechOpen

intechopen.com

Built by scientists, for scientists

Meet the editors

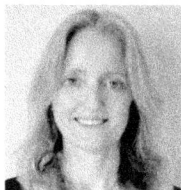

Marisa Domingues dos Santos, M. D., Ph.D., specializes in Colorectal Surgery and holds a Doctorate in Medical Sciences. She was a specialist at the College of General Surgery and the College of Clinical Nutrition of the Order of Doctors. She coordinates functions for the Reference Center for Rectal Cancer Treatment at the Centro Hospitalar Universitário de Santo António. She was the Head of the Colorectal Surgery Unit in the Department of Surgery and served as Emergency Team Leader at the Centro Hospitalar Universitário de Santo António. She is a Full Professor in the Integrated Master's in Medicine at the Institute of Biomedical Sciences Abel Salazar (ICBAS), University of Porto. She is a member of UMIB – the Multidisciplinary Unit for Biomedical Research - in the Oncology Research Group (MiO) and the Laboratory for Integrative and Translational Research in Population Health (ITR). She is also a member of the Scientific Council of the Institute of Public Health of the University of Porto.

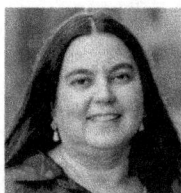

Donzília Sousa Silva, M. D., M. Sc., F. A. C. S., is a Portuguese general surgeon with expertise in hepatobiliary and pancreatic surgery, as well as liver and pancreas transplantation. She began her career as an Attending Surgeon in the Hepatobiliary and Pancreatic Unit and Liver and Pancreas Transplantation of the Centro Hospitalar Universitário de Santo António, in Porto, Portugal, where she has been working since 2007. In 2016, she became a Consultant Surgeon. She served as Head of the Hepatobiliary and Pancreatic Unit from 2017 to 2023 and has been Emergency Team Leader since 2017. She has been the Head of Clinical Governance since 2023, an Advisor to the Director of the Surgery Clinic since 2024, and an Assistant Director of the Transplantation Centre since 2024. She is an Invited Assistant Professor of Surgery at the Institute of Biomedical Sciences Abel Salazar (ICBAS), University of Porto. She obtained a Master's Degree in Organ Donation in 2010 and is currently a Ph.D. student in the field of Pancreas Transplantation.

Contents

Preface

Elective Surgery – Challenges and Practice around the World is a book that explores some of the innovations in modern surgery, their potential challenges, and the field's expected future directions. It reflects how the field continues to evolve rapidly, and how minimally invasive techniques, such as laparoscopic and robotic procedures, are gaining ground.

Written by international experts, this book is divided into five chapters and addresses hot topics in modern surgery that have had a significant impact on clinical practice.

The introductory chapter traces the evolution of surgery, highlighting technological advances, global perspectives, and patient-centered approaches that drive excellence, safety, and innovation in modern elective surgical practice.

The second chapter demonstrates how artificial intelligence is transforming robotic colorectal surgery by highlighting and augmenting reality as a key visualization technique. This tool enhances decision-making, thereby improving precision, safety, and outcomes.

The following chapter presents the innovative repair of advanced pelvic organ prolapse using an anchorless vaginal implant, highlighting surgical and technological advancements.

The fourth chapter discusses minimally invasive techniques for large suprarenal masses, illustrating the field's continuous evolution.

The purpose of the last chapter is to grow awareness of gender dysphoria, the importance of multidisciplinary care in transgender surgery, and the various technical options, particularly male-to-female genital reconstruction.

I consider this book a significant tool for enhancing global surgical knowledge, as it provides insights into practices, encourages discussion, highlights innovative methods, and promotes equitable surgical outcomes worldwide. The intention is to empower healthcare professionals to develop their expertise, achieve better patient outcomes, and collaborate globally.

Marisa Domingues dos Santos
ICBAS – School of Medicine and Biomedical Sciences,
University of Porto,
Porto, Portugal

Colorectal Surgery Unit, Clinic of Surgery,
Centro Hospitalar Universitário de Santo António (CHUdSA),
Portugal

Oncology Research Group, UMIB—Unit for Multidisciplinary
Research in Biomedicine,
University of Porto,
Porto, Portugal

ITR—Laboratory for Integrative and Translational Research
in Population Health,
Porto, Portugal

Donzília Sousa Silva
University of Porto,
Porto, Portugal

Chapter 1

Introductory Chapter: Elective Surgery – Navigating Challenges and Achieving Excellence

Donzília Sousa Silva and Marisa Domingues dos Santos

1. Introduction

It is widely accepted that the medical terminology has its roots in the ancient Greek and Latin. Surgery, however, has not born as a Greek word. The origin of the word surgery comes from the Latin *chirurgia*. The corresponding Greek term is *chirourgiki*, derived from *cheir* and *ergon*, literally meaning "hand and action," that is the action made by hands. Surgery has come a long way since the days of Hippocrates when operations were often deemed to be the last resort and conservative practices were preferred before reaching for the knife [1, 2]. Since then, surgery has navigated through revolutionary waters, faced many challenges, crossed numerous barriers, seen huge paradigm shifts, and reached the significant advances in knowledge and technologies, in its relentless pursuit for excellence.

The future of surgery is likely to be shaped by the continued advancements in technology, including the improvement of techniques, advent of artificial intelligence, machine learning, and personalized medicine. The surgical community must be prepared and remain committed to addressing the challenges and ethical issues that will arise, ensuring a promising future for surgery [3, 4].

"Elective Surgery: Challenges and Practice Around the World" is an invaluable resource to improve surgical knowledge, offering critical insights into worldwide practices, encouraging discussion, and highlighting the innovative methods and perspectives in the field of elective surgery.

2. History of surgery

Surgery has born in the earliest days of human civilization. Over the centuries, significant advancements - spanning the Middle Ages, the Renaissance, and modern times - have transformed surgical methods and our understanding of them [5]. While early civilizations laid the foundation for understanding the human body, its functions, and anatomy, later generations refined these concepts, shaping modern medical theories. Key milestones, such as the introduction of anesthesia, antiseptic techniques, and modern surgical education along with notable techniques improvements, impacted on the evolution of surgical practice and the advancements that led to the establishment of surgery as a highly specialized medical discipline [6, 7].

IntechOpen

3. Evolution of surgery

From the seventeenth century onward, surgery underwent the significant advancements driven by scientific discoveries and technological innovations. From a very rudimentary origin, surgery became increasingly specialized. In the late nineteenth and early twentieth centuries, new fields emerged, and the development of imaging technologies improved surgeons' ability to diagnose and manage conditions with greater accuracy. The advent of laparoscopic and robotic-assisted surgical techniques, in the late twentieth century, further revolutionized the field. Minimally invasive techniques reduced recovery times, minimized scarring, and improved patient outcomes and satisfaction. Today, robotic surgery enables unprecedented precision, allowing complex procedures to be performed with minimal human error [6].

The landscape in surgery is ever evolving, driven by the impetus of technological innovations. Numerous tools have merged to enhance our surgical expertise: advanced imaging technologies, minimally invasive surgery, telemedicine and remote monitoring, intelligent surgical instruments, artificial intelligence and machine learning, augmented and virtual reality, 3D printing in surgical planning, bioprinting, nanorobotics, and holographic displays. Advances in the field of surgical education and training, the establishment of checklists and protocols, a multidisciplinary culture, patient-centered approaches, and implementation of precision medicine and genomics allowed surgeons to navigate challenges and achieve excellence.

4. Book scope

Medical books can be defined based on their contents, which demonstrates differences as for the audience it addresses [8]. "Elective Surgery: Challenges and Practice Around the World" is a book that encompasses key innovations in modern surgery, their potential challenges, and the expected future directions for the field. Based on a multidimensional approach, it aims to provide valuable insights for surgeons and other clinicians, trainees, academic, and healthcare stakeholders, fostering a deeper understanding of the contemporary landscape of surgery. By sharing diverse perspectives from around the world, it serves as a comprehensive and educational resource, fostering a deeper understanding of the complexities and advancements in the field [4, 8, 9].

The book chapters travel along hot topics of modern surgery. By addressing the application of artificial intelligence in robotic colorectal surgery, it is explained how artificial intelligence can help in solving problems and making decisions, enhancing precision, safety, and outcomes. Augmented reality, as a novel data visualization tool, is a promising approach to increasing decision-making efficiency and effectiveness, enhancing knowledge conveying and comprehension [10]. The introduction of innovative devices and techniques is explored in chapter about the repair of advanced pelvic organ prolapse using an anchorless vaginal implant. The nowadays undeniable benefits of minimally invasive surgery are the topic under debate in the management of large suprarenal masses. The rise in social awareness of gender dysphoria has led to an increased recognition of the medical and surgical needs of the transgender population [11]. This kind of surgical approach remains sparsely available so implications and management will be described in detail on a dedicated chapter. Male-to-female genital reassignment surgery in gender dysphoria typifies the relevance of multidisciplinary approach.

The future of surgery will likely involve a continued emphasis on technological innovation, interdisciplinary collaboration, and the application of new knowledge to improve the patient care [12]. By encompassing a wide range of best practices within the ever-changing realm of modern surgical care, this book attempts to reach the state-of-the-art methods that collectively methodically improve the patient outcomes, and elucidate a diverse array of practices that seek to introduce new paradigms of surgery, emphasizing technological progress, patient-centered approaches, and global viewpoints. In the ever-evolving landscape of surgical care, this book's content serves as a guide for stakeholders striving to understand better and implement safe and efficient surgical procedures in various healthcare environments [13].

5. Future directions

Today, surgery continues to evolve, supported by cutting-edge technology and a greater understanding of human biology. From robotic-assisted procedures to regenerative medicine, the future of surgery promises even greater opportunities for innovation and improved patient care [5].

6. Conclusion

"Elective Surgery: Challenges and Practice Around the World" is a book that invites us to enrich our surgical knowledge to understand and manage complex scenarios, exploring the advent and implementation of new tools and technologies to improve the surgical outcomes.

Author details

Donzília Sousa Silva* and Marisa Domingues dos Santos
Santo António University Hospital Centre, Santo António Local Health Unit and School of Medicine and Biomedical Sciences, University of Porto, Porto, Portugal

*Address all correspondence to: donziliasousasilva@gmail.com

IntechOpen

References

[1] Soutis M. Ancient Greek terminology in pediatric surgery: About the word meaning. Journal of Pediatric Surgery. 2006;**41**(7):1302-1308. DOI: 10.1016/j.jpedsurg.2006.03.011

[2] Thurston LL. The history of surgery. In: Fisher R, Ahmed K, Dasgupta P, editors. Introduction to Surgery for Students. Cham: Springer; 2017. DOI: 10.1007/978-3-319-43210-6_1

[3] Haque A, Karcioglu O, Islam SB. Innovations and challenges in modern surgical practices. Asia Pacific Journal of Surgical Advances. 2024;**1**(1):1-3. DOI: 10.70818/apjsa.2024.v01i01.01

[4] Ethan A. Navigating surgical challenges: Updates in general surgery techniques and strategies. Multidisciplinary Journal of Instruction. 2021;**3**(1):94-102

[5] Rangelova D, Atanasov T. Surgery in the middle ages: Henri de Mondeville, Guy de Chauliac and Inventariumsive Chirurgia magna. Journal of Emergency Medicine. 2021;**24**(2):107-112

[6] Vretenarova T, Atanassov T, Todorova K. Surgery—From the barber-surgeon era to modern times. Bulgarian Society of Medical Sciences Journal. 2025;**7**:e153453. DOI: 10.3897/bsms.7.153453

[7] Gawande A. Two hundred years of surgery. The New England Journal of Medicine. 2012;**366**(18):1716-1723. DOI: 10.1056/NEJMra1202392. Erratum in: The New England Journal of Medicine. 2012; 367 (6): 582

[8] Kendirci M. How to write a medical book chapter? Turkish Journal of Urology. 2013;**39**(Suppl. 1):37-40. DOI: 10.5152/tud.2013.052

[9] Thurston LL. In: Martellucci J, Dal Mas F, editors. Towards the Future of Surgery. Cham: Springer; 2023. DOI: 10.1007/978-3-031-47623-5

[10] Zheng M, Lillis D, Campbell AG. Current state of the art and future directions: Augmented reality data visualization to support decision-making. Visual Informatics. 2024;**8**(2):80-105. DOI: 10.1016/j.visinf.2024.05.001

[11] Chen ML, Reyblat P, Poh MM, Chi AC. Overview of surgical techniques in gender-affirming genital surgery. Translational Andrology and Urology. 2019;**8**(3):191-208. DOI: 10.21037/tau.2019.06.19

[12] Bobadea S, Asutkar S. Current trends and future directions in surgery: A brief scoping review. Multidisciplinary Reviews. 2024;**8**(1):2025028. DOI: 10.31893/multirev.2025028

[13] Hussain A, Kakakhel M, Ashraf M, Shahab M, Ahmad F, Luqman F, et al. Innovative approaches to safe surgery: A narrative synthesis of best practices. Cureus. 2023;**15**(11):e49723. DOI: 10.7759/cureus.49723

Chapter 2

Artificial Intelligence in Robotic Colorectal Surgery

Thalia Petropoulou, Kyriacos Evangelou and Aphrodite Fotiadou

Abstract

Artificial intelligence (AI) is a growing computer science branch focused on developing systems capable of performing human intelligence-requiring tasks, such as problem-solving and decision-making. AI has made significant strides in medicine and is currently a part of diagnostics, predictive analysis, and clinical decision support. Its applications in surgery have resulted in robotic-assisting platform development, greater precision enablement, human error reduction, and surgical outcome enhancement. Augmented reality (AR) further upgraded these benefits by improving intraoperative visualisation and assisting in complex anatomical plane and structure navigation. AI can revolutionise colorectal surgery by addressing the complexity of colorectal resections and tackling the rising incidence and mortality rates of colorectal cancer (CRC). Surgical efficacy and patient outcomes are ameliorated through the facilitation of tumour detection, anatomical mapping, and surgical precision (AI) and the improvement of real-time visualisation using anatomical patient-specific 3D models (AR). This chapter highlights the latest advancements in AI-assisted robotic-assisted colorectal surgery (RAS) and showcases our pioneering work regarding the world's first live AI-assisted AR colorectal surgery with instrument de-occlusion. This significant step forward in surgical innovation is a springboard to further incorporate advanced technologies into colorectal surgery, refine and standardise AR integration, improve anatomical modelling, and expand the role of AI in RAS.

Keywords: robotic surgery, colorectal surgery, colorectal cancer, artificial intelligence, AI-assisted surgery, augmented reality, AR surgery, instrument segmentation, instrument de-occlusion, surgical innovation, right hemicolectomy

1. Introduction

Colorectal cancer (CRC) is the third most common and the second leading cause of cancer-specific mortality, with over 936,000 deaths worldwide in 2023 [1]. Approximately 21% of CRC cases are diagnosed at stage IV (metastatic) and have poor prognosis (15% at 5 years) [2]. Its incidence is increasing in developed countries, which shift towards Westernised lifestyles; diet was associated with more than one-third of CRC-related fatalities in 2019 [3].

Screening and treatment advances have improved overall CRC survival to 60–65% (5-year) in high-income countries. Early detection through colonoscopy and annual

IntechOpen

clinical examination is vital to reduce overall mortality [4–8]. Advances in novel diagnostic markers have reformed risk stratification and screening, while ongoing research into targeted and immunological therapies can further improve outcomes in advanced cases [9–13].

Although surgery remains the gold standard for localised and resectable CRC, it carries significant risks that can prolong postoperative hospitalisation and predispose to death, such as infection, haemorrhage, and anastomotic leakage. Minimally invasive techniques such as laparoscopic and robotic-assisted surgery (RAS) are therefore becoming increasingly common and can reduce complications, accelerate recovery, and improve outcomes [11, 14].

RAS offers numerous benefits for both patients and surgeons; it enables magnified, high-definition, stereoscopic 3D visualisation of intricate anatomical structures and dexterous articulated instrument manipulation with a preternatural range of motion, even in anatomically challenging sites. Tremor filtration, motor scaling, and surgeon fatigue and discomfort are minimised, ensuring enhanced accuracy, while smaller incisions limit blood loss and minimise scarring. Hereby, patients benefit from accelerated recovery, reduced postoperative pain, and lower complication risk [15, 16].

AI has revolutionised surgery and is currently evolving for colorectal RAS; preoperatively, it can improve surgical planning based on individual patient anatomy and risk factors. Intraoperatively, AI assists real-time decision-making by facilitating the visualisation of critical structures (nerve, vessel, ureter identification) and obviating the risk of injuring them. Augmented reality (AR) integration into surgery is one of the latest and most promising advancements of AI in surgery and the focal point of exploration of this chapter.

2. Applications of AI in general and CRC surgery

2.1 Development of AI

Artificial intelligence (AI) is a branch of computer science revolving around the development of systems that can perform complex tasks that typically require human intelligence (problem-solving, learning, reasoning, perception, and language understanding). AI technologies use algorithms, data processing, and pattern recognition to simulate human-like cognitive functions, enabling machines to adapt to new inputs, make decisions, and improve performance over time. Examples of AI applications include speech recognition, machine learning, robotics, and autonomous systems, all designed to mimic or enhance human abilities [1, 17].

The development of AI spans several decades, as it was officially conjoined at the Dartmouth Conference in 1956. Early AI focused on symbolic reasoning, logic-based systems, and problem-solving, but progress was slow due to limited computational power. In the 1980s, the field advanced with the introduction of expert systems, which used rule-based programming to mimic human decision-making in specialised areas. However, the real leap in AI followed the rise of machine learning in the 1990s and early 2000s [18].

Machine learning and neural networks (NN), in particular, allowed AI systems to learn from large datasets and improve over time. This shift was powered by the growth of computing power, the availability of big data, and advancements in algorithms. In recent years, deep learning (DL), a subset of machine learning (ML) involving multi-layered NN, has pushed AI to new heights, driving applications like image and speech recognition, natural language processing, and autonomous systems. Groundbreaking AI technologies such as reinforcement learning, generative models, and AI-powered robotics have further expanded its capabilities, enabling it to handle complex, real-world tasks [19].

Nowadays, AI development continues to accelerate through research in areas like explainable AI, ethical AI, and general AI, aiming to render systems more transparent, fair, and adaptable across a wide range of domains.

2.2 AI in colorectal cancer diagnosis

AI is transforming CRC diagnosis by improving the accuracy, speed, and efficiency of screening, detection, and decision-making processes [17].

AI-powered tools enhance the accuracy of detecting polyps and early-stage cancers during colonoscopy and identifying abnormalities that might be missed by the human eye [20]. This allows for earlier detection and improved patient prognosis. AI algorithms also analyse vast amounts of patient data, helping physicians make more informed decisions regarding diagnosis, risk stratification, and personalised treatment plans [21].

Additionally, AI-driven screening methods, such as virtual colonoscopy and image analysis, provide non-invasive options that enhance screening accessibility and efficiency and ultimately elevate early detection rates while reducing mortality [22].

2.3 Applications of AI in CRC treatment and surgery

The contribution of AI in CRC treatment pivots on personalising treatment plans [21]; this is primarily translated into effect assessment and pathological complete response (pCR), tumour regression grading (TRG), and neoadjuvant rectal score (NAR) prediction for (neo)adjuvant chemo-radiotherapy. Targeted therapy research can benefit from novel target identification, computer-aided drug (CAD) design approaches, gene expression and drug effect monitoring, medicine precision, and tumour target segmentation [17].

Visualisation is the centrepiece of AI in colorectal surgery, as the development of techniques such as fluorescence imaging and laser speckle contrast imaging (LSCI) represents a significant milestone [1]; the former most commonly employs indocyanine green (ICG) dye to assess anastomosis perfusion, lymph node detection, and even ureter identification, whose injury is a main concern. LSCI analyses the blurring effect of the speckle pattern following laser light illumination and helps investigate tissue perfusion in real-time without the need for a fluorophore or delay between contrast injection and blood flow evaluation. AI can provide objective measurements in both cases and even real-time anatomical structure identification through AR patient-specific 3D-model overlay intraoperatively **(Figure 1)** [23].

Perhaps the most important breakthrough brought upon colorectal surgery is the establishment of robotic platforms and, hence, the opportunity to develop simulation training programmes for new surgeons and residents. Hands-on training involves virtual (VR) instead of augmented reality training and can offer hand-eye coordination improvement, learning curve improvement, procedural familiarity in a risk-free environment before performing actual surgeries, real-time feedback from proctors even in other countries at the time, opportunities to practice rare or complex cases,

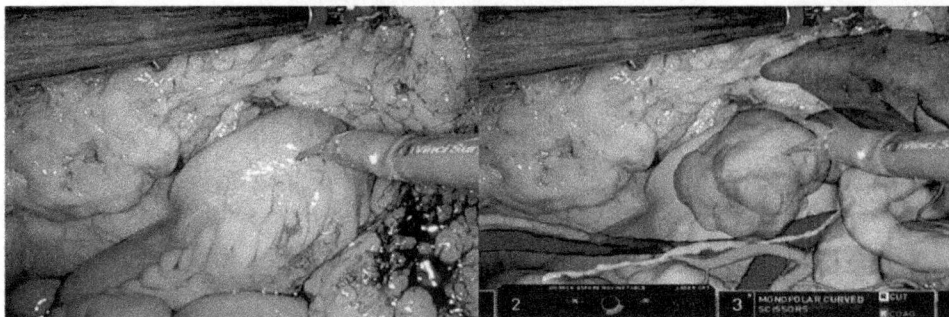

Figure 1.
Intraoperative view of the surgical field as displayed on the robotic monitor before (left) and after (right) the AR 3D patient-specific model overlay.

and personalised training programmes based on skill levels [24]. On this account, more and more fundings are being awarded for new AI model development for robotic surgical skill training, such as the very recent £25,000 grant to the School of Biomedical Engineering and Imaging Sciences of King's College by the Royal College of Surgeons of England [25].

3. Anatomical segmentation and augmented reality (AR) in surgery

3.1 Image segmentation from multi-slice (CT/MRI) scans

A technique called image segmentation is applied for 3D-model fabrication of patient anatomy and is broadly classified as manual (MS), semi-automated (SAS), or fully automated (FAS) [26]. Although the former is the gold standard and generates the most accurate models, it is remarkably time-consuming and impractical. SAS is the optimal fusion of the former and latter that leverages both human expertise and computational efficiency to streamline the process by improving efficiency, accuracy, repeatability, and workflow. There are ongoing attempts to refine availability and develop novel FAS algorithms.

FAS faces multiple challenges and is currently not possible with acceptable accuracy; anatomical variations, structural complexity, image quality (noise and artefacts), lack of context understanding, limited training data for rarer conditions, low contrast between structures, and lack of dynamical adaptation to new data reduce its applicability to real-world clinical settings. For CRC, advancing DLM, such as convolutional NN using large datasets, is emerging as a promising endeavour to ameliorate and standardise FAS [27].

3.2 First documented application and benefits of AR in general surgery

The first documented application of AR in general surgery was reported in late 2004 by an IRCAD-EITS (European Institute of Telesurgery) team [28]; a 45-year-old man with a 1-cm right adrenal gland Conn adenoma underwent laparoscopic right adrenalectomy, and the authors remarked that AR helped determine the correct dissection planes and the location of the tumour, adjacent organs, and vessels.

Intraoperative AR has been gaining ground in many subspecialties, such as urological, hepatic, and colorectal surgery [29].

AR in surgery offers multiple benefits that improve surgical outcomes; spatial perception is improved, and superfluous tissue manipulation that increases the risk of injury is avoided. This decreases the overall operative time and ensures patient safety by minimising human error. AR also enhances surgical education by offering realistic simulations and helping young surgeons practice complex techniques in a risk-free environment.

3.3 AR in robotic-assisted colorectal surgery

It was not until early 2021 that the first case of robotic CME in Europe with AR (proximie) overlay of the 3D-reconstructed vascular anatomy was reported by our team [30]. CME + D3-lymphadenectomy were successfully performed with the real-time guidance of an intuitive proctor from London, and final pathology revealed a 9-cm T3N0 right colon tumour with 48 harvested LNs and an intact mesocolon.

A new era of AR-assisted robotic surgery is dawning as AI-system initiatives are announced around the world. Perhaps one of the most interesting projects is the AI-powered surgical visualisation tool EUREKA α™ that received regulatory approval in Japan this spring [31]; the Arnaut Inc.-developed tool is equipped with precision mapping technology that allows for intraoperative real-time connective tissue, nerve, dissection plane, blood vessel, and organ highlight and overlay.

3.4 Challenges of AR integration in colorectal surgery

Standardising AR in colorectal surgery is considerably more demanding than in other surgical subspecialties due to the anatomical peculiarity of the colon. Its convoluted and tubular shape is constantly changing positions and complicates intraoperative visualisation and mapping compared to solid and fixed organs (e.g., kidney, liver, prostate). The colon is more mobile during surgical manipulation than, e.g., the kidneys (fixed inside Gerota's fascia); its dynamic shape makes it more difficult for AR to maintain its accuracy due to unpredictable changes in shape and position.

Additionally, morphometric and spatial lymphovascular anatomy variations are common (as opposed to, e.g., the lungs and liver), and multiple critical structures such as the ureters, nerves, and pelvic organs surround the colon and rectum; it is therefore imperative to align 3D models with regard to the vessels and not the colon and rectum, unlike the rest of the organs.

4. Instrument occlusion and de-occlusion during AR RAS

4.1 Addressing the issue of instrument occlusion during AR RAS

Although AR during RAS permits 3D-model superimposition over manipulated tissue [32], these models frequently overlay non-organic items such as cutting instruments and engender a hazardous intraoperative environment [33]. There have been multiple attempts to tackle this problem, albeit unsuccessful and infeasible [34–36]. What is needed is to automatically identify instruments and prioritise their visibility by eliminating obscuring 3D-model overlays (**Figure 2**).

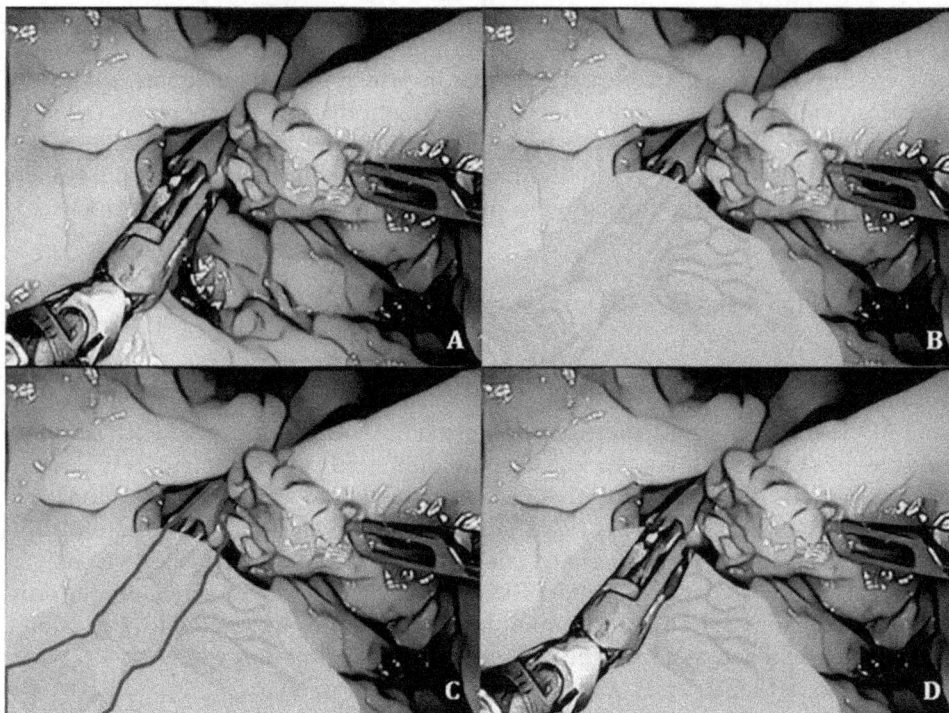

Figure 2.
Schematic representation of the instrument occlusion by overlaid 3D models during the AR surgery issue. (A) Intraoperative view during a robotic right hemicolectomy before AR model integration. (B) Instrument occlusion by the AR-generated 3D models of the underlying tumour (green area) and blood vessels (red). (C): Occluded and non-occluded instrument identification. (D): De-occlusion through segmentation.

4.2 First-in-human real-time AI-assisted instrument de-occlusion during AR RAS

The first in-human real-time AI-assisted instrument de-occlusion during AR RAS was reported in late 2023 in *Healthcare Technology Letters* by Jasper Hofman and Pieter De Backer of the ORSI Academy as co-first authors [37]. The team developed software and implemented hardware for a robust real-time binary segmentation pipeline for instrument de-occlusion; a 31,812-image dataset from 100 full-length robotic partial nephrectomies was used for algorithm training (75.7%), validation (14.3%), and testing (10.0%) with a combination of a Feature Pyramid Network (FPN) with EfficientNetV2 encoder backbone. Their hardware solution consisted of a NVIDIA Clara AGX developer kit as embedded computing architecture, and an integrated DELTA-12G-elp-key card was used for live video capture. CT- or MRI-based 3D models were preoperatively fabricated using the Materialise Mimics 3D Medical Imaging Processing Software, and the setup was applied in three different hospitals during a partial nephrectomy, a migrated endovascular stent removal, and a liver metastasectomy.

Notwithstanding its training on partial nephrectomy instrument segmentation exclusively, the algorithm had demonstrated good general implementation, having achieved a test set accuracy of more than 98%. Conversion from PyTorch to TensorRT reduced interference time from 40.5 to 5.1 seconds without sacrificing accuracy, while the pipeline effectively de-occluded instruments with a per-frame latency of 13 milliseconds. The perceived end-to-end latency was satisfactory for real-time applications, as indicated by qualitative surgical feedback.

4.3 World's first live AI-assisted AR colorectal surgery with instrument de-occlusion

To our knowledge, we have performed the world's first live AI-assisted AR colorectal surgery with instrument de-occlusion at the Euroclinic General Hospital of Athens. The patient was a 45-year-old man with a 12 cm ascending colon tumour invading the lateral abdominal wall with suspicious paraaortic lymph nodes on CT. Triple-phase 1 mm CT images were employed to segment the anatomy using manual and semi-automated methods (**Figure 3**).

The segmentation resulted in the fabrication of an individualised 3D anatomical model that would later be integrated during surgery (**Figure 4**).

Robotic CME with D3 and paraaortic lymphadenectomy were planned, and AR was selected to ensure major structure (SMA, SMV) injury prevention, gastrocolic trunk of Henle identification, and peripancreatic LN clearance.

During surgery, the 3D model was manually aligned with the patient's anatomy and displayed over the endoscopic image. A binary segmentation model ensured that the overlay was transparent for non-organic elements, preventing instrument occlusion (**Figure 5**).

This AI-assisted AR pipeline was deployed in real-time using NVIDIA Clara AGX hardware and displayed in TilePro in the surgeon console (**Figure 6**).

A proof-of-concept livestream was set up with a LiveArena capture card and a laptop running Microsoft Teams. Our experience will be presented orally during the 15th Clinical Robotic Surgery Association (CRSA) Worldwide Congress on Gems and

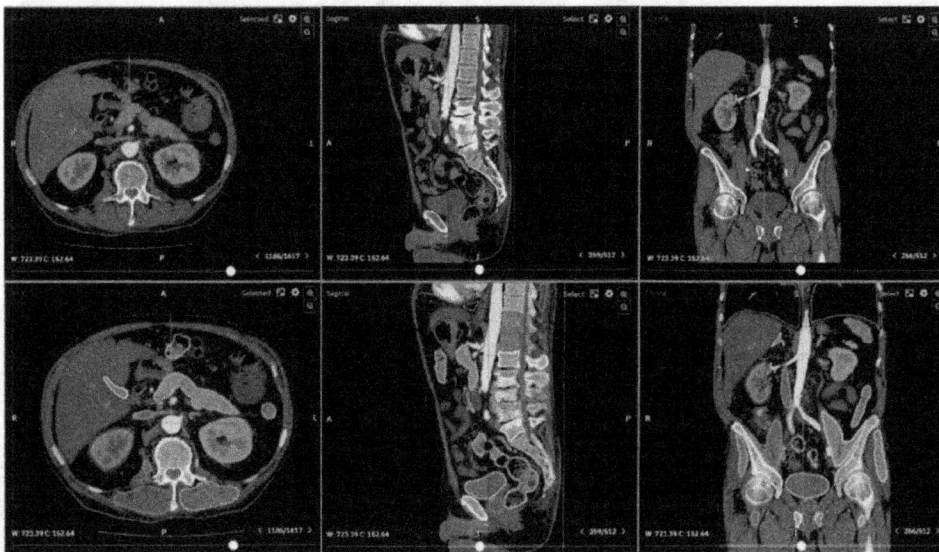

Figure 3.
Manual and semi-automated anatomy segmentation outcomes from triple-phase 1 mm CT images. Upper row: raw CT scan images. Bottom row: segmented CT scan images. Left column: axial section. Middle column: sagittal section. Right column: coronal section.

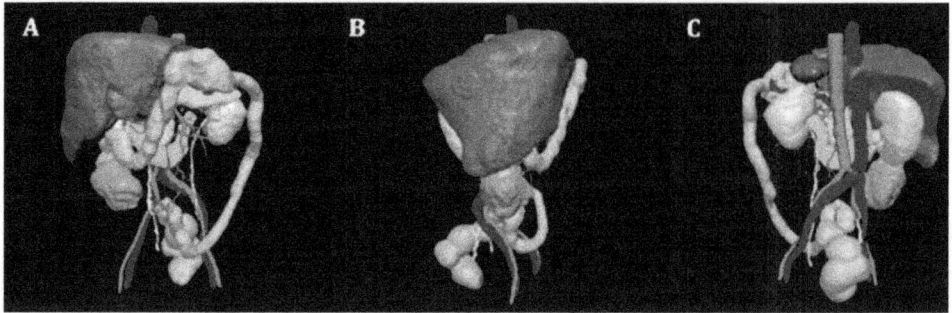

Figure 4.
Patient-specific 3D anatomical model fabricated from segmented CT images illustrating the right colon tumour (pink). (A): anterior view. (B): right lateral view. (C): posterior view.

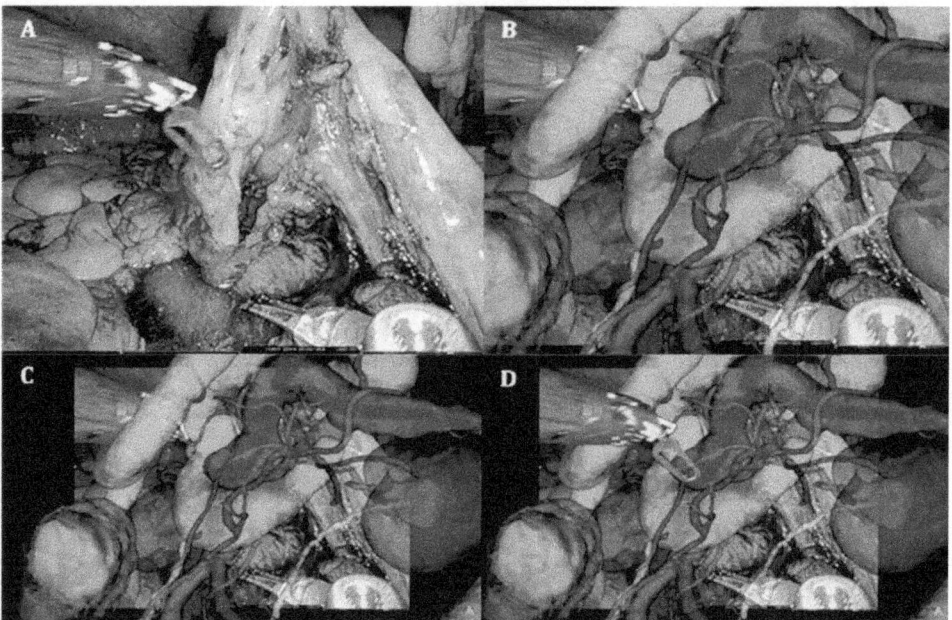

Figure 5.
Instrument occlusion and de-occlusion during the surgery. (A): raw view of the surgical field. (B): 3D-model overlay over both instruments. (C): Instrument identification and segmentation. (D): instrument de-occlusion.

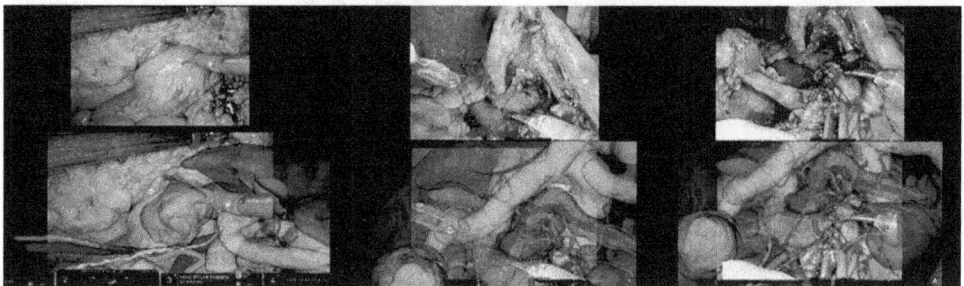

Figure 6.
Intraoperative view of the surgical field as displayed on the robotic monitor. Upper row: raw visualisation. Bottom row: post-3D-model overlay and instrument de-occlusion surgical field view.

Artificial Intelligence in Robotic Colorectal Surgery
DOI: http://dx.doi.org/10.5772/intechopen.1009893

Hints from the International Experts on Clinical Robotics and Surgical Innovation, which will take place in Rome from November 21 to 23, 2024.

5. Future perspectives on AI and AR in robotic colorectal surgery

The successful execution of the world's first live AI-assisted AR colorectal surgery with instrument de-occlusion by our team marks a pivotal moment in surgical innovation that paves the way for the integration of advanced technologies (AI) in colorectal surgery and the wider adoption of AR.

AI-driven personalised treatment plans will be a key area of future development; AI systems could analyse large volumes of patient-specific data (including genomics, medical history, and imaging results) to tailor highly personalised surgical approach and technique plans and minimise complications while improving outcomes in such varying anatomy and cancer, such as in colorectal resections.

Enhanced intraoperative AI assistance might represent another upcoming major advancement; providing real-time decision-making support, analysing intraoperative data and offering recommendations on optimal resection techniques or strategies to minimise surrounding healthy tissue damage can remarkably aid surgeons, who could apply immediate adjustments to improve patient safety and outcomes.

It is speculated that semi-autonomous and fully-autonomous robotic systems might be an exciting area of potential development; independently performing routine or repetitive tasks such as suturing or tissue dissection with minimal human oversight, although a long-term goal at the moment, can allow surgeons to focus on more complex and critical aspects of the procedure.

6. Conclusions

The integration of artificial intelligence (AI) and augmented reality (AR) into colorectal surgery can redefine the landscape of surgical advancement, especially regarding robotic-assisted surgery (RAS). AI is capable of detecting robotic surgical instruments, and real-time AR can even be combined with browser livestreaming. We have demonstrated that intraoperative AI-assisted AR RAS is feasible, safe, and effective for colorectal cancer surgery; nevertheless, manual registration to the anatomy is necessary due to non-deformable 3D models and lack of tissue tracking and espouses a notable barrier that calls for dedicated research to overcome and fully release the potential of semi- to fully-autonomous AI. As these technologies continue to evolve, their potential to revolutionise RAS in colorectal cancer (CRC) and enhance training for future surgeons is immense.

Acknowledgements

We would like to thank the ORSI academy for providing the 3D colorectal anatomy models for intraoperative AR overlay.

Conflict of interest

The authors declare no conflict of interest.

Notes/thanks/other declarations

The authors declare no additional notes or other declarations.

Author details

Thalia Petropoulou[1,2]*, Kyriacos Evangelou[3] and Aphrodite Fotiadou[4]

1 Department of Robotic Colon and Rectal Surgery, Euroclinic General Hospital of Athens, Athens, Greece

2 Aretaieio Hospital, National and Kapodistrian University of Athens, Athens, Greece

3 National and Kapodistrian University of Athens, Athens, Greece

4 Department of General, Visceral and Transplantation Surgery, University Hospital of Heidelberg, Heidelberg, Germany

*Address all correspondence to: thalia_pet@hotmail.com

IntechOpen

References

[1] World Health Organization (WHO). Colorectal Cancer; 2023. Available from: https://www.who.int/news-room/fact-sheets/detail/colorectal-cancer [Accessed: September 20, 2024]

[2] Lingam G, Shakir T, Kader R, Chand M. Role of artificial intelligence in colorectal cancer. Artificial Intelligence in Gastrointestinal Endoscopy. 2024;5(2):90723. DOI: 10.37126/aige. v5.i2.90723

[3] Liang Y, Zhang N, Wang M, Liu Y, Ma L, Wang Q, et al. Distributions and trends of the global burden of colorectal cancer attributable to dietary risk factors over the past 30 years. Nutrients. 2023;16(1):132. DOI: 10.3390/nu16010132

[4] Heisser T, Hoffmeister M, Tillmanns H, Brenner H. Impact of demographic changes and screening colonoscopy on long-term projection of incident colorectal cancer cases in Germany: A modelling study. The Lancet Regional Health - Europe. 2022;30(20):100451. DOI: 10.1016/j. lanepe.2022.100451

[5] Siegel RL, Wagle NS, Cercek A, Smith RA, Jemal A. Colorectal cancer statistics, 2023. CA: a Cancer Journal for Clinicians. 2023;73(3):233-254. DOI: 10.3322/caac.21772

[6] Rawla P, Sunkara T, Barsouk A. Epidemiology of colorectal cancer: Incidence, mortality, survival, and risk factors. Przeglad Gastroenterologiczny. 2019;14(2):89-103. DOI: 10.5114/pg.2018.81072

[7] Bretthauer M, Løberg M, Wieszczy P, Kalager M, Emilsson L, Garborg K, et al. Effect of colonoscopy screening on risks of colorectal cancer and related death. The New England Journal of Medicine. 2022;387(17):1547-1556. DOI: 10.1056/NEJMoa2208375

[8] American Cancer Society. Colorectal Cancer Early Detection, Diagnosis, and Staging, Last Revised: January 29, 202. Available from: https://www.cancer.org/cancer/types/colon-rectal-cancer/detection-diagnosis-staging/acs-recommendations.html [Accessed: September 20, 2024]

[9] Gmeiner WH. Recent advances in therapeutic strategies to improve colorectal cancer treatment. Cancers. 2024;16:1029. DOI: 10.3390/cancers16051029

[10] Pathak PS et al. State-of-the-art Management of colorectal cancer: Treatment advances and innovation. American Society of Clinical Oncology Educational Book. 2024;44:e438466. DOI: 10.1200/EDBK_438466

[11] Krieg A, Kolbe EW, Kaspari M, et al. Trends and outcomes in colorectal cancer surgery: A multicenter cross-sectional study of minimally invasive versus open techniques in Germany. Surgical Endoscopy. 2024;38(11):6338-6346. DOI: 10.1007/s00464-024-11210-1

[12] Chan DLH, Segelov E, Wong RS, Smith A, Herbertson RA, Li BT, et al. Epidermal growth factor receptor (EGFR) inhibitors for metastatic colorectal cancer. Cochrane Database of Systematic Reviews. 2017;6(6):CD007047. DOI: 10.1002/14651858.CD007047

[13] Deniz C, Guven, Kavgaci G, Erul E, Syed MP, Magge T, et al. The efficacy of immune checkpoint inhibitors in microsatellite stable colorectal cancer:

A systematic review. The Oncologist. 2024;**29**(5):e580-e600. DOI: 10.1093/oncolo/oyae013

[14] Pak H, Maghsoudi LH, Soltanian A, Gholami F. Surgical complications in colorectal cancer patients. Annals of Medicine and Surgery. 2020;**55**:13-18. DOI: 10.1016/j.amsu.2020.04.024

[15] Shah J, Vyas A, Vyas D. The history of robotics in surgical specialties. American Journal of Robotic Surgery. 2014;**1**(1):12-20. DOI: 10.1166/ajrs.2014.1006

[16] Reddy K, Gharde P, Tayade H, Patil M, Reddy LS, Surya D. Advancements in robotic surgery: A comprehensive overview of current utilizations and upcoming Frontiers. Cureus. 2023;**15**(12):e50415. DOI: 10.7759/cureus.50415

[17] Yin Z, Yao C, Zhang L, Qi S. Application of artificial intelligence in diagnosis and treatment of colorectal cancer: A novel Prospect. Frontiers in Medicine. 2023;**8**(10):1128084. DOI: 10.3389/fmed.2023.1128084

[18] Delipetrev B, Tsinarakii C, Kostić U. Historical Evolution of Artificial Intelligence. Luxembourg: EUR 30221EN, Publications Office of the European Union; 2020. DOI: 10.2760/801580

[19] Sengar SS, Hasan AB, Kumar S, et al. Generative artificial intelligence: A systematic review and applications. Multimedia Tools and Applications. arXiv. 2024. arXiv:2405.11029. DOI: 10.1007/s11042-024-20016-1

[20] Joseph J, LePage EM, Cheney CP, Pawa R. Artificial intelligence in colonoscopy. World Journal of Gastroenterology. 2021;**27**(29):4802-4817. DOI: 10.3748/wjg.v27.i29.4802

[21] Maleki Varnosfaderani S, Forouzanfar M. The role of AI in hospitals and clinics: Transforming healthcare in the 21st century. Bioengineering (Basel). 2024;**11**(4):337. DOI: 10.3390/bioengineering11040337

[22] Mitsala A, Tsalikidis C, Pitiakoudis M, Simopoulos C, Tsaroucha AK. Artificial intelligence in colorectal cancer screening, diagnosis and treatment. A New Era. Current Oncology. 2021;**28**(3):1581-1607. DOI: 10.3390/curroncol28030149

[23] Simion L, Ionescu S, Chitoran E, Rotaru V, Cirimbei C, Madge OL, et al. Indocyanine green (ICG) and colorectal surgery: A literature review on qualitative and quantitative methods of usage. Medicina (Kaunas, Lithuania). 2023;**59**(9):1530. DOI: 10.3390/medicina59091530

[24] Piozzi GN, Subramaniam S, Di Giuseppe DR, Duhoky R, Khan JS. Robotic colorectal surgery training: Portsmouth perspective. Annals of Coloproctology. 2024;**40**(4):350-362. DOI: 10.3393/ac.2024.00444.0063

[25] King's College London. Research Team Awarded Funding to Develop New AI Models for Robotic Surgical Skills Training [Internet]; 2024. Available from: https://www.kcl.ac.uk/news/research-team-awarded-funding-to-develop-new-ai-models-for-robotic-surgical-skills-training [Accessed: September 25, 2024]

[26] Luzon JA, Kumar RP, Stimec BV, Elle OJ, Bakka AO, Edwin B, et al. Semi-automated vs. manual 3D reconstruction of central mesenteric vascular models: The Surgeon's verdict. Surgical Endoscopy. 2019;**34**(11):4890-4900. DOI: 10.1007/s00464-019-07275-y

[27] Cao K, Yeung J, Arafat Y, Qiao J, Gartrell R, Master M, et al. Using a new

artificial intelligence-aided method to assess body composition ct segmentation in colorectal cancer patients. Journal of Medical Radiation Sciences. 2024;**71**(4):519-528. DOI: 10.1002/jmrs.798

[28] Marescaux J, Rubino F, Arenas M, Mutter D, Soler L. Augmented-reality–assisted laparoscopic adrenalectomy. Journal of the American Medical Association. 2004;**292**(18):2211. DOI: 10.1001/jama.292.18.2214-c

[29] Fu J, Rota A, Li S, Zhao J, Liu Q, Iovene E, et al. Recent advancements in augmented reality for robotic applications: A survey. Actuators. 2023;**12**(8):323. DOI: 10.3390/act12080323

[30] Petropoulou T, Polydorou A, Amin S. First robotic CME in Europe with augmented reality tools. Techniques in Coloproctology. 2021;**25**(7):887-888. DOI: 10.1007/s10151-021-02413-y

[31] Anaut Announces Japanese Regulatory Approval of AI-Powered Surgical Visualization Tool, Eureka α [Internet]; 2024. Available from: https://www.biospace.com/anaut-announces-japanese-regulatory-approval-of-ai-powered-surgical-visualization-tool-eureka-%CE%B1 [Accessed: September 9, 2024]

[32] Seetohul J, Shafiee M, Sirlantzis K. Augmented reality (AR) for surgical robotic and autonomous systems: State of the art, challenges, and solutions. Sensors. 2023;**23**(13):6202. DOI: 10.3390/s23136202

[33] Qian L, Wu JY, DiMaio SP, Navab N, Kazanzides P. A review of augmented reality in robotic-assisted surgery. IEEE Transactions on Medical Robotics and Bionics. 2020;**2**(1):1-16. DOI: 10.1109/tmrb.2019.2957061

[34] Kutter O, Aichert A, Bichlmeier C, Traub J, Heining SM, Ockert B, et al. Real-time volume rendering for high quality visualization in augmented reality. In: International Workshop on Augmented Environments for Medical Imaging Including Augmented Reality in Computer-Aided Surgery (AMI-ARCS 2008). New York, USA: Navis Publications; Sep 2008. pp. 104-113

[35] Frikha R, Ejbali R, Zaied M. Handling occlusion in augmented reality surgical training based instrument tracking. In: 2016 IEEE/ACS 13th International Conference of Computer Systems and Applications (AICCSA). Agadir, Morocco: IEEE; 2016. pp. 1-5

[36] De Backer P, Van Praet C, Simoens J, Peraire Lores M, Creemers H, Mestdagh K, et al. Improving augmented reality through deep learning: Real-time instrument delineation in robotic renal surgery. European Urology. 2023;**84**(1):86-91. DOI: 10.1016/j.eururo.2023.02.024

[37] Hofman J, De Backer P, Manghi I, Simoens J, De Groote R, Van Den Bossche H, et al. First-in-human real-time AI-assisted instrument deocclusion during augmented reality robotic surgery. Healthcare Technology Letters. 2023;**11**(2-3):33-39. DOI: 10.1049/htl2.12056

Chapter 3

Repair of Advanced Pelvic Organ Prolapse Using an Anchorless Vaginal Implant

Zviya Fridman-Kogan, Naama Marcus and Gil Levy

Abstract

Pelvic organ prolapse (POP) is a common condition that is treated by surgical reconstruction of the connective support structures in the pelvis. Although surgical POP repair using trans-vaginal mesh (TVM) provides good anatomical results, it is known to cause serious complications, and clinical studies support the conclusion that the need for mesh anchoring is the main reason for these complications. The self-retaining support (SRS) implant was designed to address the root causes of current mesh-related complications, as it is an anchorless TVM device. It exploits the advantages of POP meshes while eliminating the need for mesh fixation, and there is a documented body of evidence demonstrating its safety and effectiveness. This chapter discusses surgical outcome criteria for POP repair and existing TVM solutions, followed by a discussion of the anchorless SRS implant. A review of the published studies demonstrating safety and effectiveness of the SRS implant is presented, followed by a discussion of SRS surgical technique and complications management. Given that the anchorless SRS implant addresses the complications associated with anchored TVMs, its utility for the safe and effective treatment of POP should be considered as part of the surgical alternatives for POP repair.

Keywords: pelvic organ prolapse, trans-vaginal mesh, self-retaining support, anchorless implant, anatomical success, subjective success, neo-fascia

1. Introduction

Pelvic organ prolapse (POP), a common condition among women, is caused by damage to the pelvic organs' supporting structures, including ligaments, fasciae, and muscles [1]. Symptomatic POP is treated by surgical reconstruction of the connective support structures. Various surgical approaches have been proposed over time based on our understanding of the structure of pelvic organ support and the risk profile of the corrective procedures.

Three levels of pelvic organ support were described by DeLancey in 1992, namely Level I support (suspension), in which the section of the vagina adjacent to the cervix

IntechOpen

is suspended by long connective tissue fibres of the upper paracolpium, Level II support (attachment), in which the paracolpium becomes shorter in the middle section of the vagina and attaches the vaginal wall laterally to the pelvic walls, and Level III support (fusion), in which the vagina near the introitus is fused laterally to the levator ani muscles and posteriorly to the perineal body [2]. Based on these levels, surgical techniques were developed to restore each level of support separately, i.e. site-specific repair. Damage to Level II support in the anterior compartment was traditionally repaired by anterior colporrhaphy. Improved restoration of Level II support was achieved by the introduction of synthetic materials, which augmented or replaced the damaged connective tissue. Simultaneously, it was demonstrated that restoring Level I (apical) support was key to achieving surgical success [3], and implant anchoring techniques were therefore modified to achieve repair of both Level I and Level II support. This was achieved by extending the mesh fixation points towards the sacrospinous ligaments. Trans-vaginal meshes (TVMs) therefore gained traction for POP repair.

Historically, surgical POP repair using TVMs was found to provide good anatomical results [4, 5]. However, the use of TVMs was brought into question due to reports of intra- and post-operative complications, which included organ perforation, bleeding, mesh erosion, mesh contraction, and pain [5, 6]. In 2008, the United States FDA issued a public health notification alerting health practitioners to the complications associated with transvaginal placement of surgical meshes to treat POP [7]. This was followed by a safety communication in 2011, which stated that transvaginal POP repair with mesh led to serious complications that were not rare, and questioned whether this procedure was more effective than traditional non-mesh repair [8]. In 2016, the FDA reclassified surgical mesh for transvaginal repair of POP as class III devices [9] and in 2019 ordered all manufacturers of surgical mesh intended for transvaginal POP repair to stop selling and distributing their products, as they did not demonstrate reasonable assurance of safety and effectiveness [10]. In addition to the FDA, the European Association of Urology (EAU), the European Urogynecological Association (EUGA), and Sheffield Teaching Hospitals National Health Service (NHS) Foundation Trust recommended in 2017 that synthetic mesh should only be used in complex POP cases with recurrent prolapse in the same compartment [11]. Following these events, the use of TVMs for POP surgery was notably reduced, and native tissue repair (NTR) or sacrocolpopexy became the preferred approaches for POP repair, despite having sub-optimal long-term success rates [12]. Although NTR is safe, it was initially reported to have a success rate over time of only ~50% based on anatomical results [13], which was then "improved" to ~73% compared to TVM procedures [14] by changing the definition of success to include subjective success (i.e. patient satisfaction). Abdominal approaches such as sacrocolpopexy and lateral suspension are more invasive and complicated, have comparable safety issues to TVMs, and might not suit all patients due to the higher risk for patients with surgical comorbidities [15]. There is therefore a need for improved transvaginal approaches for POP repair that incorporate the effectiveness of TVM approaches without the safety concerns.

An alternative approach for addressing the safety concerns of surgical mesh for POP repair is the use of an anchorless mesh device, as clinical studies support the conclusion that the need for mesh anchoring may be the main reason for the complications encountered with mesh kits used for POP repair (see Section 3.2 for further details) [16]. An anchorless approach would allow the benefits and effectiveness of mesh implants to be retained, while eliminating complications associated with their use. This chapter describes the anchorless self-retaining support (SRS) solution in the context of surgical outcome criteria and existing approaches for POP repair with TVM. At the end of the chapter, the authors discuss SRS implantation surgical technique and complications management [17].

2. Pelvic organ prolapse—Surgical outcome criteria

There has been much debate over the years regarding the definition of success following POP surgical repair. The NIH and International Continence Society (ICS) uses the pelvic organ prolapse quantification (POP-Q) system [18] and define pure objective anatomical success after surgical intervention as Ba < −1 cm, i.e. ICS POP-Q grade ≤ 1 [19]. However, the pelvic floor disorder network (PFDN) proposed less stringent criteria for success—an anatomical outcome where the leading edge of anterior prolapse is at or above the hymen, i.e. Ba ≤ 0 cm [20]. The 2009 study performed for the PFDN, which analysed 18 different surgical success definitions in patients who underwent abdominal sacrocolpopexy, found that cure rates that used less stringent anatomical criteria for all segments or that considered only support of the vaginal apex were more consistent with subjective cure rates. Subjective cure was defined as absence of vaginal bulge symptoms, assessed using the following questions in the pelvic function distress inventory (PFDI): "Do you usually have a sensation of bulging or protrusion from the vaginal area?" and "Do you usually have a bulge or something falling out that you can see or feel in the vaginal area?". The PFDN study also concluded that subjective cure was significantly associated with the patients' evaluation of overall improvement, which is not the case with anatomical success alone [20]. They thus sought to consider patient satisfaction when determining the success of POP surgery, which would ensure that the benefits were justified in comparison with the risks. The FDA consequently adopted this approach, focusing on symptom relief criteria.

While it is clearly important to consider both objective (anatomical) and subjective (patient experience) outcomes, it is recommended to assess these outcomes individually. The authors believe that this is not achieved using the approach adopted by the FDA, as the PFDN success criterion of Ba ≤ 0 cm practically merges objective *and* subjective considerations. The addition of pure subjective results (i.e. absence of vaginal bulge symptoms) then serves as a further bias towards the subjective considerations. While this seems to be an adequate bias, it may serve as a double-edged sword, considering the patients' long-term overall quality-of-life. A symptomatic woman undergoing surgical reconstruction surgery that reduces her leading edge prolapse from +1 to 0 cm will be considered a successful technique. Long-term follow-up with a change of the prolapsed leading edge in 1 cm from ba = 0 to ba = +1 will disqualify the technique as inadequate allowing initial approval of surgical techniques with weak anatomical outcomes to be approved. In addition, if anatomical success is defined as non-bulging of the leading edge (i.e. Ba ≤ 0 cm) and failure is considered a bulge (i.e. Ba > 0 cm), then the difference between anatomical failure and success is reduced to a few millimetres during the Valsalva manoeuvre. This minor difference between failure and success can impact the evaluation of surgical techniques. More stringent anatomical results are undoubtedly better than less stringent anatomical outcomes and are not expected to negatively impact subjective results (**Figure 1**). Achieving more stringent criteria for anatomical success at the time of POP surgery also allows for longer term efficacy, as should deterioration occur post-surgery due

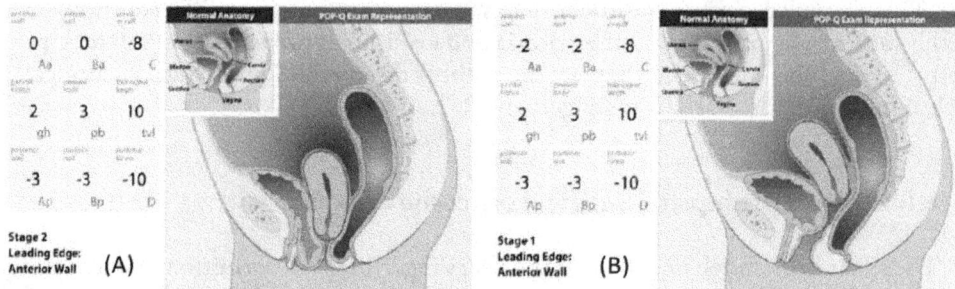

Figure 1.
Different objective success criteria: (A) Less stringent anatomical success criteria (PFDN)—Ba ≤ 0 cm. (B) More stringent anatomical success criteria (NIH)—Ba < −1 cm, which allows minor anatomical deterioration over time without subjective impact.

to mechanical stresses and ageing, a change from Ba −2 to −1 cm is not anticipated to have a significant impact on symptoms or the patient's subjective assessment/satisfaction. This would therefore likely reduce the need for repeat surgical procedures, whereas deterioration from Ba 0 to 1 cm would most probably lead to re-treatment.

Studies that compare results when using the PFDN/FDA anatomical outcome versus NIH anatomical outcomes have demonstrated that the different outcome definitions lead to different conclusions regarding superiority or non-inferiority of POP repair interventions [21]. It is thus essential that the definition of success following POP repair surgery is carefully considered. The recommended approach is to use a composite primary endpoint that includes both pure anatomical and pure subjective success criteria which are assessed in parallel, but independently of each other. With this approach, the NIH anatomical success criteria (Ba < −1 cm) should be used, and subjective success should be defined as responses of "no" or "not at all" to question number 3 of the PFDI Short Form 20 (PFDI-20) questionnaire, i.e. "Do you usually have a bulge or something falling out that you can see or feel in your vaginal area?". A composite primary endpoint using more stringent anatomical success criteria provides a higher standard for success compared to the criteria suggested by the PFDN and adopted by the FDA.

3. Current anchor-based mesh solutions

3.1 Types of mesh solutions

There are numerous types of TVM solutions, which differ by their anchoring/fixation method to pelvic structures. These anchor-based mesh solutions include Boston Scientific's "Uphold" kit utilising two anchoring points (withdrawn from the market), Coloplast's "Restorele®" kit (withdrawn from the market), Promedon's "Calister®" kit, and Neomedic's "Surelift®" kit, all having four anchoring points, and AMI's "InGYNious®" kit with six anchoring points. In addition, various mesh materials can be used, including allografts (such as cadaveric fascia or dura mater), xenografts (such as porcine or bovine), autografts (such as fascia lata or rectus fascia), and synthetic meshes (such as non-absorbable polypropylene [PP] or polyvinylidene fluoride [PVDF] meshes, absorbable meshes, or a combination of both) [11].

3.2 Anchored mesh complications

It is well known that TVM solutions are accompanied by intra- and post-operative complications and safety concerns, as has been acknowledged by various medical associations, including the International Urogynecological Association (IUGA), the American Urogynecologic Society (AUGS), the EAU, and the EUGA [11, 22, 23]. Complications may include chronic pain and dyspareunia, mesh erosion, and mesh contraction [7, 8, 24]. Management of mesh-related complications can be complex, involving various surgical procedures from partial to complete vaginal mesh excision, depending on the specific situation [22].

3.2.1 Chronic pain and dyspareunia

Mesh sheets are implanted between the bladder and vagina and are therefore subject to anatomical forces in addition to the forces arising from scar tissue accumulation. These forces may cause the mesh to bunch and fold in on itself. Such mesh contraction and bunching can cause nerve entrapment and/or excessive tension on the fixated mesh arms, both of which might lead to pain. Indeed, it is well documented that mesh folding and contraction is the main reason for chronic pelvic pain and dyspareunia (**Figure 2**) [16], with partial removal of the mesh at the fixation points and a reduction in mesh tension resolving symptoms in 90% of patients [25]. It has also been shown that procedures that use polypropylene mesh which is not firmly fixated, such as graft augmented colporrhaphy (mesh reinforced NTR) and Johnson and Johnson's "Prosima" kit, do not involve pelvic pain [26]. It is therefore evident that the need to anchor TVMs into the pelvic structures is the main reason for the development of chronic pain after POP repair.

3.2.2 Mesh erosion and mesh contraction

Mesh folding may be an important factor that contributes to mesh exposure, as a folded mesh does not lie flat against the vaginal wall, and may therefore impede

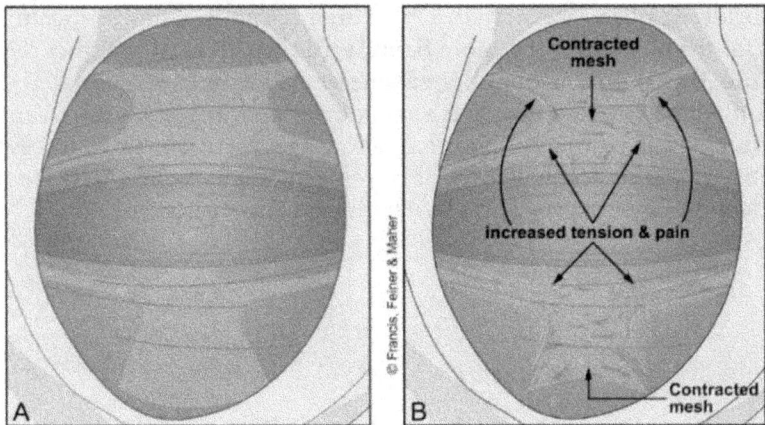

Figure 2.
(A) Layout of anterior vaginal mesh with four arms and posterior vaginal mesh with two arms at implantation, and (B) after the body of the mesh has contracted by 30%. In (B), increased tension is indicated by narrowing of the arms, and areas of pain by curved lines. Illustration: Stephen Francis. Copyright ©2009, Francis, Feiner, and Maher (Source: Feiner and Maher [16]).

healing at the incision site [27]. Indeed, mesh folding was identified in nine out of 13 patients (69%) who suffered from vaginal mesh exposure [27]. Eliminating mesh folding and bunching may therefore reduce exposure through the vaginal incision and may lessen the rate of mesh erosion. Nevertheless, implantation and securing techniques used with anchored mesh kits (i.e. fixation of standalone meshes at two, four, or six corners in the pelvis) do not ensure that the mesh is placed in a tension-free, flat, non-folded fashion, despite this being emphasised by the manufacturer's instructions and training programmes [16]. Even when the mesh is placed in a flat and tension-free configuration during the surgical procedure, dynamic pressures and accumulating scar contraction forces may still result in mesh contraction and folding over time.

In addition to mesh folding, anchoring has been investigated in the context of mesh erosion. A retrospective study that proposed a different surgical fixation technique for a mesh product with a high rate of erosion (4–19%) found that altering the fixation points and technique alone could reduce the erosion rate to ~1% [28]. This study thus demonstrates that anchoring can play an important role in mesh erosion.

3.2.3 Pore size and pore configuration changes

After implantation of a TVM, the porous area of the mesh creates a scaffold for the ingrowth of new fibrous tissue [29]. Inflammatory processes are initiated as part of mesh incorporation into the tissue, including fibrogenesis, which is mediated by fibroblast proliferation (fibroplasia). This process is accompanied by angiogenesis, collagen synthesis, and collagen maturation (cross linking) for scar tissue formation [30].

Scarring is associated with contraction of the wound area, which leads to 20–40% shrinkage of the mesh 10 months post-implantation [31]. The porous nature of the mesh—microporous (small-pore) versus macroporous (large-pore)—plays a signifi-cant role in this process. Microporous mesh leads to a significantly lower deposition of healthy type 1 collagen compared to macroporous mesh [29]. Microporous mesh is thus associated with "bridging fibrosis", which leads to increased mesh stiffness, as opposed to macroporous mesh in which the greater distance between the pores can resist the "bridging fibrosis". Therefore, macroporous mesh is more biocompatible and allows for the formation of a more flexible scar, which better mimics the native tissue (**Figure 3**) [29]. In addition, pore diameters of <1 mm are associated with an enhanced inflammatory response that accompanies poor tissue ingrowth and fibrotic encapsulation [32]. In contrast, large pores allow neovascularization, access for leuko-cytes and macrophages, and ingrowth of fibroblasts and collagen. All this contributes to lower infection rates and supports incorporation into the tissue [33].

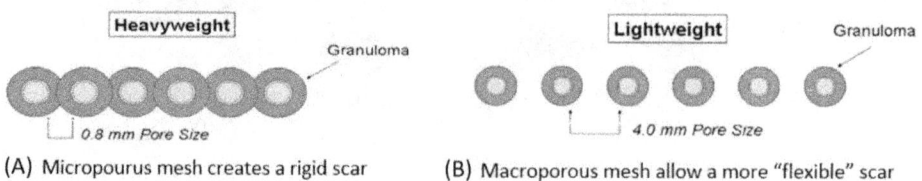

(A) Micropourus mesh creates a rigid scar   (B) Macroporous mesh allow a more "flexible" scar

Figure 3.
(A) Microporous and (B) macroporous mesh. Scar plate formation occurs with microporous (small-pore) mesh due to bridging fibrosis, while macroporous (large-pore) mesh allows growth of healthy type 1 collagen between the filaments (Source: Cobb et al. [29]).

Of note, after implantation, anchored TVM meshes are thought to be more likely to lose pore configuration than hernia meshes [34]. Any mechanical force load onto the mesh dramatically decreases the size of the pore [35, 36]. For example, a study by Barone et al. that investigated porosity and pore diameter of four synthetic mesh products using uniaxial testing found that an application of 5 N led to a decrease in porosity of as much as 87% [36]. With regard to currently available transvaginal mesh products, total pore collapse is expected at some load, and it is therefore important to consider the maintenance of pore diameter in the design of mesh products [36].

3.3 Use of mesh solution for pelvic organ prolapse repair

The use of TVM solutions for POP repair has been the subject of much debate over the years. Historically, the use of TVM for the surgical treatment of POP was found to provide good anatomical results [4, 5]. However, in 2019 the FDA ordered mesh manufacturers to stop selling devices for transvaginal repair of POP, as data were not provided to support a favourable benefit-risk profile compared to NTR at 12 months [10, 37]. More recently, Nager et al. published 5-year results of the Study of Uterine Prolapse Procedures—Randomised Trial (SUPeR Trial), which compared sacrospinous hysteropexy with graft (polypropylene mesh) to vaginal hysterectomy with bilateral uterosacral ligament suture apical suspension (native tissue vaginal hysterectomy) [38]. The study found that mesh hysteropexy resulted in a lower composite failure rate than vaginal hysterectomy through 5 years, supporting the superiority of vaginal mesh hysteropexy procedures [38]. Therefore, the authors suggested that the FDA ban on these products should be reconsidered [38]. In addition, Kahn et al. published 3-year results from a prospective, parallel cohort trial that compared TVM with NTR for the treatment of POP, demonstrating that TVM was non-inferior in the primary efficacy outcome and superior in the secondary efficacy outcome (the primary outcome was determined by the FDA, but was criticised as it included anatomical outcome measures that were the same as the inclusion criteria) [21]. With regard to serious adverse events, TVM was found to be as safe as NTR [21]. The results from both these studies suggest that vaginal mesh repair has sustained long-term efficacy. In particular, the use of an anchorless device would allow the benefits and efficacy of mesh implants to be retained, while eliminating the complications associated with their use.

4. The self-retaining support anchorless solution

4.1 The anchorless solution theory

The SRS implant is an anchorless transvaginal implant that is designed to mimic the physiological pubocervical fascia, thereby restoring pelvic organs to their anatomical and functional location. The device, which is manufactured by Lyra Medical Ltd., comprises a solid, flexible, polymer, U-shaped frame, and a titanised, ultra-light (16 g/m^2), extra-thin (65 μm fibre), AMID Type 1 polypropylene mesh (**Figure 4**). The implant's flexible frame ensures that the mesh layer remains flat and in the desired location, eliminating the need for fixation, while the mesh serves as a scaffold for the creation of a support structure. The SRS implant thereby provides "trampoline-like" support to the prolapsed anterior and apical compartments. Following DeLancy's levels of support, Level II support is provided by creating an anchorless

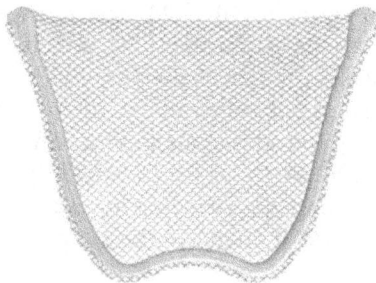

Figure 4.
Self-retaining support implant.

neo pubocervical fascia that imitates the physiological supporting structures, while extending the depth of the device to the level of the ischial spines provides additional Level I support. In addition, the anatomical location of the SRS bridge at the bladder neck provides Level III support, thus affording complete tri-level support of the anterior and apical compartments in one device. Taken as a whole, the SRS implant exploits the advantages of commercially available POP meshes while eliminating the need for mesh fixation.

The SRS implant was designed to address the root causes of current mesh-related complications (**Video 1**, https://drive.google.com/file/d/1sSqRfKEIGpsY_ GDxORu3TbiHb2c-NGsr/view?usp=sharing). The implant inhibits mesh erosion, as the solid frame retains mesh tension and prevents it from folding, as was demonstrated in a cadaver study which confirmed that the device is maintained in the appropriate anatomical position [39]. The frame also acts as an opposing mechanical force that prevents mesh contraction, maintaining the implant's flat configuration and the macroporous mesh structure. By maintaining a tension-free, flat orientation, the implant also prevents pelvic pain. The risk of dyspareunia is likewise reduced, as the SRS implant provides bladder support without causing tension across the vagina. In addition, the SRS implant reduces the risk of bleeding and organ perforation during the surgical procedure, as SRS implantation does not require blind insertion of surgical instruments such as trocars or anchoring instruments. The design of the SRS implant with lack of fixation points thus prevents the pain and complications that are common with current anchored mesh kits.

4.2 Safety and effectiveness of self-retaining support implantation

The safety and effectiveness of the SRS implant has been demonstrated in multiple published studies. In the initial stages of development, a cadaver study was performed to assess the feasibility and anatomical landmarks of the SRS device [39]. Dissections of two cadavers in whom the SRS device had been implanted transvaginally confirmed that the device was located in an appropriate anatomical position, at a safe distance from vital neurovascular structures in the pelvis [39].

Following the cadaver study, a prospective, multicentre, international study of 20 women with at least second-degree anterior compartment prolapse, with/without apical prolapse, was performed to evaluate the feasibility, safety, and cure rate of POP repair with the SRS implant [40]. This initial study suggested that the SRS implant could be used safely and effectively in clinical settings, with optimal anatomical and subjective cure at 2 years and no intra- or immediate post-operative adverse events

[40]. Thereafter, a second protocol with 50 women was initiated, and combined results for the 70 women, all of whom underwent POP surgery with the SRS implant, were analysed [41]. Average surgical time for device implantation was 24.7 minutes, with no intra-operative complications. At last follow-up (mean follow-up time post-surgery of 27.7 months), POP-Q staging of the anterior compartment demonstrated 57 (81%) patients at grade 0, nine (13%) at grade 1, and four (6%) at grade 2 [41]. Thus, anatomical success rate (grade 0 and grade 1) in the 70 patients was 94%. In addition, notable anatomical changes were demonstrated at points Aa, Ba, and C, with mean (range) measurements from baseline to last follow-up of 2.0 (−1 to 3) cm to −2.9 (−3 to −1) cm at point Aa, 3.1 (−2 to 6) cm to −2.8 (−3 to −1) cm at point Ba, and 0.4 (−8 to 6) cm to −6.8 (−10 to 1) cm at point C [41]. Subjectively, based on the PFDI-20 questionnaire, 97% of patients were cured, and there were no reports of chronic dyspareunia in the 38 patients who completed the relevant questionnaire (pelvic organ prolapse/urinary incontinence sexual questionnaire [PISQ12]) [41]. Among the 70 patients who received SRS implants, two (3%) underwent partial frame resection. The first patient presented with vaginal discharge and was diagnosed with frame erosion 8 months post-surgery, following which the eroded part was resected. This was possibly caused using a large size frame, given that this was the only patient in whom a large size was used. The mesh size was selected intraoperatively by the surgeon. The surgeon had to confirm that the solid frame does not apply any pressure on the vaginal wall prior to closure of the vaginal incision. Initially, three sizes of frames were developed: large, medium, and small. Intraoperative observation revealed that the medium size was suitable for most patients and thus became the most commonly utilised. No comparative study was conducted between the different frame sizes; rather, the selection of the medium frame size was based on the surgeon's experience. The second patient was diagnosed with voiding dysfunction at the 12-month follow-up visit, which was assumed to be caused by pressure from the solid bridge, and the sub-urethral frame bridge was therefore resected. In addition, two patients (3%) developed de-novo stress urinary incontinence (SUI) and underwent a mid-urethral sling procedure [41]. At follow-up, two patients (3%) had recurrent prolapse, one of whom was symptomatic and received treatment, with no instances of mesh erosion or chronic pelvic pain [41]. The expanded study of 70 patients thus demonstrated that the SRS implant could be an effective and safe treatment for POP, providing 94% objective and 97% subjective cure, with only 2 patients (3%) requiring surgical removal of the implant frame.

These 70 patients were followed up over time, and long-term results at 36 months were available for 67 patients (median follow-up of 38.4 months) [17]. At the final visit, mean (range) post-operative Aa, Ba, and C values were −2.9 (−3 to −1) cm, −2.8 (−3 to −1) cm, and −6.9 (−10 to 1) cm, respectively, all of which were significantly different from the baseline (pre-operative) values (p < 0.05) [17]. Sixty (86%) patients were stage 0 at the final visit, six (9%) were stage 1, and four (6%) were stage 2 above the hymen (Ba < 0 cm) [17]. Thus, anatomical success was 94% based on stage 0 or 1, or 100% based on a success criterion of Ba ≤ 0 cm. Clinical outcome was not significantly impacted by body mass index, smoking, diabetes, or parity. Subjective success, which was based on question number 3 of the PFDI-20 questionnaire analysed for the index surgical compartment, reached 96% [17]. Among patients who did not undergo a concomitant posterior colporrhaphy with their SRS implantation, there was evidence of a 27% worsening of the posterior compartment prolapse [17]. During follow-up there were no cases with mesh exposure or chronic pelvic pain. In total, over the course of the 36-month study, complications included two cases of transient urinary retention, one case of minor frame exposure, one case of voiding dysfunction, and two cases of de novo SUI [17]. This study thus demonstrated that in the long term (to 36 months), SRS implantation achieves excellent subjective and objective success rates, with minimal complications.

A comparative study of the anchorless SRS implant has also demonstrated positive findings [42]. Results from SRS implantation in the 70 patients included in the above studies were retrospectively compared to results from patients undergoing anchored TVM implantation and NTR. Patients in all three cohorts presented with anterior and/or apical prolapse stage 2 or higher and were followed up for a comparable time, though there were differences in age and parity between the cohorts [42]. Compared to the anchored TVM (n = 106) and NTR (n = 49) groups, the SRS group (n = 70) demonstrated significantly better post-operative Aa measurements (−2.31 cm, −1.07 cm and −2.87 cm, respectively; $p < 0.05$) and Ba measurements (−2.08 cm, −0.87 cm and −2.81 cm, respectively; $p < 0.05$) [42]. The SRS group also reported a higher mean difference improvement in PFDI-20 scores (anchored TVM group = 15.94, NTR group = 9.8 and SRS group = 49.01; $p < 0.05$) [42]. In terms of safety outcomes, the SRS group had fewer post-operative complications, less recurrent prolapse, and lower risk of revisional surgery [42]. It was thus demonstrated that compared to anchored TVM or NTR, the SRS implant more readily restored measurable parameters of anterior vaginal wall prolapse and improved quality of life [42].

An additional retrospective study was performed to summarise the surgical experience of repairing advanced POP with the SRS implant at a single university hospital [43]. Sixty women with at least second-degree vaginal anterior prolapse (with/without apical prolapse) who had undergone SRS implantation and had an increased risk of prolapse recurrence were recruited, and their medical files reviewed [43]. In addition, question number 3 of the PFDI-20 questionnaire was administered telephonically, and patients who reported a bulging sensation were referred for follow-up examination at the clinic. It was found that four (7%) women underwent reoperation due to prolapse recurrence of the posterior and vaginal apex. Six (10%) women who reported a bulging sensation telephonically had a prolapse of the posterior compartment—but not of the anterior or apical compartment treated by the SRS—upon vaginal examination [43]. The combined results of the repeat surgeries and the questionnaire demonstrated a 93% success rate for the SRS implant at a mean follow-up of 14 months [43]. No intra-operative complications were documented, with only four (7%) patients having surgical field hematomas that required conservative treatment [43]. During post-operative follow-up, one patient was found to have mesh erosion in the surgical incision that was treated vaginally with an estrogenic preparation, and one patient suffered from vaginal bleeding due to granulation tissue in the surgical incision [43]. No chronic pelvic pain, dyspareunia, dyspraxia, or other complications that required resection of the SRS implant were documented. This study thus demonstrated the safety and effectiveness of the SRS implant for women with advanced anterior and apical vaginal prolapse [43].

There is thus a documented body of evidence demonstrating the safety and effectiveness of the SRS implant for POP surgical repair. While additional, larger, randomised controlled clinical trials are required, these studies provide promising results regarding this anchorless implant. Despite the favourable safety and effectiveness profile, which demonstrates that the SRS implant addresses complications associated with TVM, official position statements regarding POP repair and mesh-related complications that have been published by the IUGA, AUGS, EAU, and EUGA do not mention the SRS device or cite these data [11, 22, 23]. These statements include recommendations to only use synthetic mesh for POP repair in complex cases with recurrent prolapse (EAU and EUGA statement) [11] and most recently (2023) to use NTR as the first-line approach for POP repair (EUGA recommendation) [23]. These recommendations may have been different had the safety and effectiveness data regarding the SRS implant been considered. In addition, the outcome statistics used in the SRS studies demonstrate the superiority of the SRS implant compared to other TVM devices. Patient selection for the SRS implant should be based on the following indications: Women for whom NTR surgical correction failed or who have risk factors that increase their likelihood of experiencing recurrence of prolapse after NTR repair will be offered the option of using a vaginal mesh implant. These risk factors are based on lifestyle conditions that lead to significant and/or chronic increases in intra-abdominal pressure. Such risk factors include occupations requiring heavy lifting (e.g. homecare work, caregiving in geriatric institutions, gardening, and kindergarten teachers) or intensive physical activities (e.g. long-distance running and high-impact sports involving jumping). Another group of women that should be considered as high risk for failure of native tissue repair are patients with high MBI (>30) secondary to chronic increase in intra-abdominal pressure and women with high parity (>4 vaginal deliveries) secondary to major obstetrics trauma/collagen damage to the pelvic organ support system. We believe that patients with contraindications for sacrocolpopexy, i.e. severe intra-abdominal adhesions secondary to multiple surgeries, or women who failed sacrocolpopexy, should be offered the option of vaginal mesh surgery although there is not enough scientific data to support it.

4.3 Surgical technique

The surgical technique for implanting the SRS device involves central dissection of the bladder from the vagina, which extends to the paravesical space for direct bilateral palpation of the ischial spines. The device is inserted between the bladder and the vaginal mucosa with the lateral arms following the anatomy of the arcustendineus-fascia-pelvis (ATFP). The connecting bridge is positioned under the pubic symphysis (**Figure 5**). Appropriate location is confirmed by visualisation of a symmetrically positioned device and a fully stretched mesh under the bladder (**Figure 6**). In cases of uterine preservation, in order to maintain the cervix positioning and prevent it from slipping underneath the implant's mesh, the inner aspect of the upper cervical lip is sutured to the middle of the proximal edge of the mesh. If there is tension on the implant, the surgeon is instructed to remove the device, extend the dissection area, and re-insert it. The vaginal incision is then closed with no tension, and vaginal packing is used for 24 hours.

Video 2 showing a live surgical procedure can be viewed at https://drive.google.com/file/d/1R-rtW4CrsemVjtTFIVPH7mhoTsJQQZGQ/view?usp=sharing.

4.4 Complications management

Complications of SRS implantation reported in a cohort of 70 patients have been minimal, including transient urinary retention, minor frame exposure, delayed voiding dysfunction, and de novo SUI [17, 41]. Surgical field hematomas requiring conservative treatment, mesh erosion (one case), and vaginal bleeding due to granulation tissue in the surgical incision (one case) have also been reported in the second cohort of patients who underwent SRS implantation [43]. Correct management of SRS complications is essential to ensure the safety of this device and improved patient outcomes.

The most important consideration pertaining to surgical complications is prevention. Correct dissection of the bladder from the vagina and ensuring that the dissection area is wide enough to accommodate the entire implant's shape and size will have the greatest impact on preventing adverse events. In addition, it is important to ensure

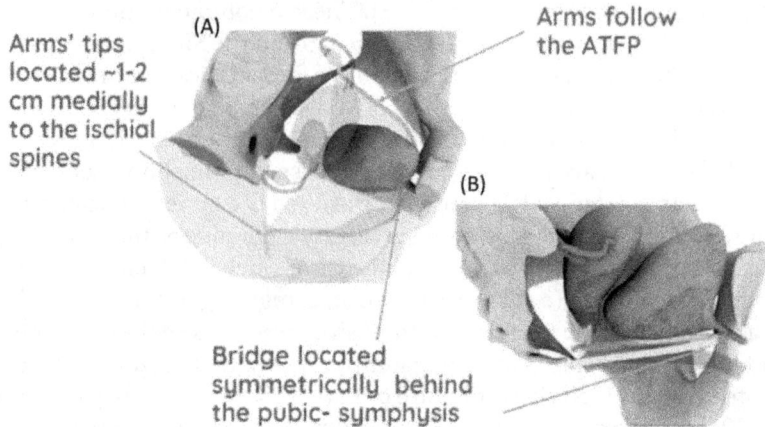

Figure 5.
SRS anatomical location—(A) top view and (B) side view.

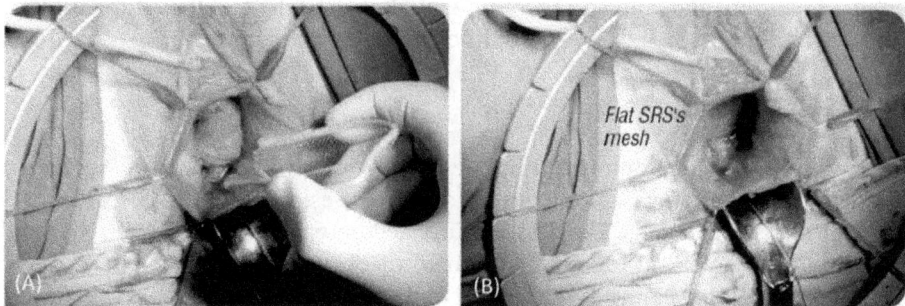

Figure 6.
(A) SRS insertion, following which (B) the implanted SRS frame retains a flat, tension-free mesh.

that the SRS implant is correctly positioned and does not apply pressure on any of the surrounding tissues, particularly the vaginal mucosa. The arm tips of the SRS implant should be located at the ischial spines, with the arms following the ATFP. The bridge of the implant should be located symmetrically at the level of the bladder neck. If there is tension on the implant at the time of the implantation procedure, the surgeon should extend the dissected area, making sure that the implant does not apply any forces on the surrounding tissue [40].

Procedures to manage possible complications are discussed below [17].

4.4.1 Frame erosion

Frame erosion is caused by insufficient dissection (para urethral and/or around the ischial spine), leading to pressure on the vaginal mucosa, which may result in extrusion of part of the frame (usually the corners of the bridge section). It is treated by resecting the exposed part of the frame under local or regional anaesthesia in an ambulatory surgical procedure (**Figure 7**). The resection involves infiltrating the mucosa around the erosion with local anaesthetic and incising the area surrounding the exposed frame (~1 cm from each side). Thereafter, the exposed frame is held with a Kelly clamp, and traction is applied in order to dissect the surrounding tissue

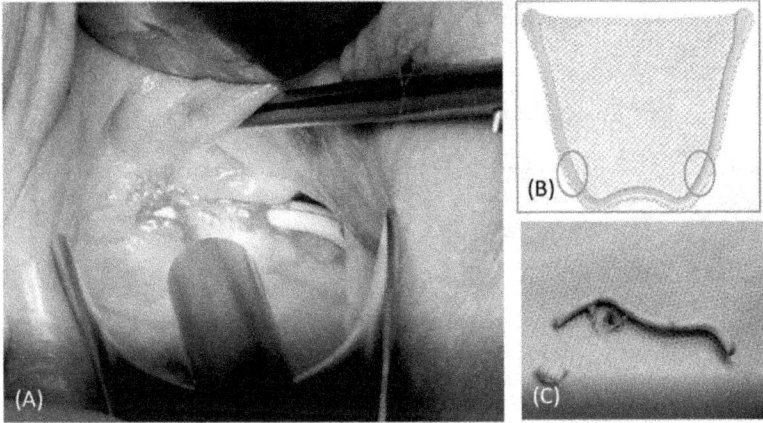

Figure 7.
(A) Frame erosion, which is treated by (B) cutting the frame ~1–1.5 cm above the bridge angle towards the arms tips in order to (C) resect the exposed part of the frame.

and expose the SRS bridge. The mesh along the bridge inner aspect is then detached using a scalpel. A cutter, preferably a curved cutter (e.g. orthopaedics bone cutter or dermatologists nail cutter), is used to cut the frame ~1–1.5 cm above the bridge angle towards the arms tips on each side. Avoiding the sharp edges of the remaining frame's arms, the inflamed mucosal edges are trimmed as needed. The incision should be closed using absorbable suture material.

4.4.2 Urinary retention

The bridge of the SRS implant was designed with a notch/curve to allow free passage of the urethra and prevent the risk of obstruction. In a proper dissection, the bridge is positioned 3–4 mm from the urethra/bladder-neck. Nevertheless, patients who undergo SRS implantation may potentially experience urinary retention, incomplete emptying, or voiding difficulties. Differential diagnoses include detrusor hypoactivity prior to surgery or wrong bridge location which causes pressure on the urethra. A video-urodynamics study or trans-perineal ultrasound is recommended to confirm the bridge location and rule out urethral obstruction. In case of unresolved urinary retention (obstructive or non-obstructive), the preferred treatment involves resection of the SRS bridge under local or regional anaesthesia as described for frame erosion.

4.4.3 Incision dehiscence

Patients with incision dehiscence present with bleeding at the surgical scar. Root causes may include anticoagulation medication, which can be a risk factor for surgical site hematoma, insufficient haemostasis of the surgical field, or insufficient dissection that causes incision closure under tension. Thus, prevention of incision dehiscence includes waiting to restart long-acting anticoagulation medication for 72 hours post-surgery (if possible), employing good surgical field haemostasis, and reducing tension on the surgical incision by sufficient dissection and tension-free approximation of the incision edges.

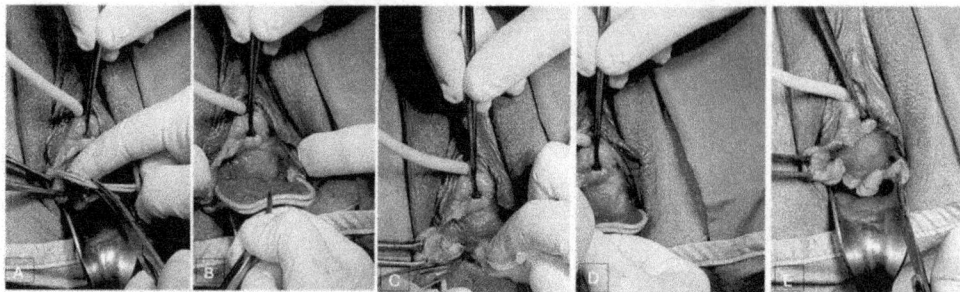

Figure 8.
Resection of the SRS implant: (A) detachment of the mesh from the SRS bridge, (B) applying pooling pressure on the frame, (C) dissection of the tissue surrounding the SRS frame, (D) detachment of the mesh from the SRS arms, and (E) complete removal of the SRS implant.

Where dehiscence is suspected, an examination of the surgical scar should be performed. Transvaginal ultrasound is also recommended to assess for hematoma. In cases of small dehiscence, conservative therapy is indicated, whereas large dehiscence and complete exposure of the implant to the vaginal cavity requires removal of the implant. Note that unlike other transvaginal implants, it is generally easier to locate the implant, as the frame acts as the implant's borderline. In cases of surgical field hematoma, it is likely that the implant has not been incorporated into the surrounding tissue, which may ease the extraction.

Steps for resection of the implant are shown in **Figure 8**. This is performed using a Kelly clamp to apply traction to the SRS exposed frame. The mesh is then freed from the surrounding tissue using blunt dissection, following which the surgical edges are trimmed, and the implant bed is washed with antiseptic solution. The incision is closed with absorbable suture material.

5. Conclusions: The future of surgical implants for the treatment of pelvic organ prolapse

POP is a common condition requiring safe and effective surgical intervention. Although the use of surgical TVM for POP repair has historically shown good results, the many intra- and post-operative complications have raised serious concerns regarding the safety of these implants. NTR is therefore used as the current standard-of-care, despite its limited efficacy. It has been demonstrated that the adverse events associated with TVMs are largely due to the need to anchor the mesh into the pelvic structure, and the anchorless concept is thus a promising alternative to traditional anchored mesh devices. The SRS implant provides long-term anatomical success and patient satisfaction, with minimal risk of morbidity or exposure and little need for re-intervention. However, studies with longer follow-up and bigger sample sizes are still required, including randomised controlled trials that compare SRS implantation with NTR to assess longer-term outcomes in patients with symptomatic anterior and apical compartment POP. Such studies should use a composite endpoint including both objective and subjective definitions of success. Given that the anchorless SRS mesh implant addresses the complications associated with anchored TVMs, its utility for the safe and effective treatment of POP is very promising.

Acknowledgements

The authors gratefully acknowledge the surgeons who contributed to the initial experience with the SRS implant, namely Dr. Anat Beck, Prof. Mauro Cervigni, Dr. Anna Padoa, Dr. Eyal Goldschmit, Prof. Alfredo Ercoli, and Prof. Zoltan Fekete.

Conflict of interest

Dr. Gil Levy initiated the development of the SRS device.

Notes

The SRS device is approved for use in countries in Europe, Israel, and Central America.

Author details

Zviya Fridman-Kogan[1], Naama Marcus[2] and Gil Levy[1]*

1 Assuta Samson University Hospital, Ashdod, Israel

2 Ziv Medical Center, Zefat, Israel

*Address all correspondence to: gille@asuta.co.il

IntechOpen

References

[1] Thakur R, Mally J, Karki S, Nijamudin, Jun WY, Hua ZX, et al. Transvaginal mesh procedures for prolapse, analyzing its outcome rates and complications-literature review. Gynecology. 2013;**1**:4. DOI: 10.7243/2052-6210-1-4

[2] DeLancey JO. Anatomic aspects of vaginal eversion after hysterectomy. American Journal of Obstetrics and Gynecology. 1992;**166**:1717-1724; discussion 1724-1728. DOI: 10.1016/0002-9378(92)91562-o

[3] Eilber KS, Alperin M, Khan A, Wu N, Pashos CL, Clemens JQ, et al. Outcomes of vaginal prolapse surgery among female Medicare beneficiaries: The role of apical support. Obstetrics and Gynecology. 2013;**122**:981-987. DOI: 10.1097/AOG.0b013e3182a8a5e4

[4] Vitale SG, Laganà AS, Gulino FA, Tropea A, Tarda S. Prosthetic surgery versus native tissue repair of cystocele: Literature review. Updates in Surgery. 2016;**68**:325-329. DOI: 10.1007/s13304-015-0343-y

[5] Maher C, Feiner B, Baessler K, Schmid C. Surgical management of pelvic organ prolapse in women. The Cochrane Database of Systematic Reviews. 2013;**4**:CD004014. DOI: 10.1002/14651858.CD004014.pub5

[6] Altman D, Väyrynen T, Engh ME, Axelsen S, Falconer C, Nordic Transvaginal Mesh Group. Anterior colporrhaphy versus transvaginal mesh for pelvic-organ prolapse. The New England Journal of Medicine. 2011;**364**:1826-1836. DOI: 10.1056/NEJMoa1009521

[7] Food and Drug Administration. FDA Public Health Notification: Serious Complications Associated with Transvaginal Placement of Surgical Mesh in Repair of Pelvic Organ Prolapse and Stress Urinary Incontinence [Internet]. 2008. Available from: https://wayback.archive-it.org/7993/20170111190506/http://www.fda.gov/MedicalDevices/Safety/AlertsandNotices/PublicHealthNotifications/ucm061976.htm [Accessed: 24 September 2024]

[8] Food and Drug Administration. UPDATE on Serious Complications Associated with Transvaginal Placement of Surgical Mesh for Pelvic Organ Prolapse: FDA Safety Communication [Internet]. 2011. Available from: https://wayback.archive-it.org/7993/20170111231226/http://www.fda.gov/MedicalDevices/Safety/AlertsandNotices/ucm262435.htm [Accessed: 24 September 2024]

[9] Food and Drug Administration. Obstetrical and Gynecological Devices; Reclassification of Surgical Mesh for Transvaginal Pelvic Organ Prolapse Repair [Internet]. 2016. Available from: https://www.federalregister.gov/documents/2016/01/05/2015-33165/obstetrical-and-gynecological-devices-reclassification-of-surgical-mesh-for-transvaginal-pelvic [Accessed: 24 September 2024]

[10] Food and Drug Administration. Urogynecologic Surgical Mesh Implants [Internet]. 2021. Available from: https://www.fda.gov/medical-devices/implants-and-prosthetics/urogynecologic-surgical-mesh-implants [Accessed: 24 September 2024]

[11] Chapple CR, Cruz F, Deffieux X, Milani AL, Arlandis S, Artibani W, et al. Consensus statement of the European Urology Association and the European

Urogynaecological Association on the use of implanted materials for treating pelvic organ prolapse and stress urinary incontinence. European Urology. 2017;**72**:424-431. DOI: 10.1016/j.eururo.2017.03.048

[12] Siddiqui NY, Grimes CL, Casiano ER, Abed HT, Jeppson PC, Olivera CK, et al. Mesh sacrocolpopexy compared with native tissue vaginal repair: A systematic review and meta-analysis. Obstetrics and Gynecology. 2015;**125**:44-55. DOI: 10.1097/AOG.0000000000000570

[13] Kontogiannis S, Goulimi E, Giannitsas K. Reasons for and against use of non-absorbable, synthetic mesh during pelvic organ prolapse repair, according to the prolapsed compartment. Advances in Therapy. 2017;**33**:2139-2149. DOI: 10.1007/s12325-016-0425-3

[14] Steures P, Milani AL, van Rumpt-van de Geest DA, Kluivers KB, MIJ W. Partially absorbable mesh or native tissue repair for pelvic organ prolapse: A randomized controlled trial. International Urogynecology Journal. 2019;**30**:565-573. DOI: 10.1007/s00192-018-3757-5

[15] Costantini E, Brubaker L, Cervigni M, Matthews CA, O'Reilly BA, Rizk D, et al. Sacrocolpopexy for pelvic organ prolapse: Evidence-based review and recommendations. European Journal of Obstetrics, Gynecology, and Reproductive Biology. 2016;**205**:60-65. DOI: 10.1016/j.ejogrb.2016.07.503

[16] Feiner B, Maher C. Vaginal mesh contraction: Definition, clinical presentation, and management. Obstetrics and Gynecology. 2010;**115**:325-330. DOI: 10.1097/AOG.0b013e3181cbca4d

[17] Levy G, Padoa A, Marcus N, Beck A, Fekete Z, Cervigni M. Surgical treatment of advanced anterior wall and apical vaginal prolapse using the anchorless self-retaining support implant: Long-term follow-up. International Urogynecology Journal. 2022;**33**:3067-3075. DOI: 10.1007/s00192-021-05045-w

[18] Madhu C, Swift S, Moloney-Geany S, Drake MJ. How to use the pelvic organ prolapse quantification (POP-Q) system? Neurourology and Urodynamics. 2018;**37**:S39-S43. DOI: 10.1002/nau.23740

[19] Weber AM, Abrams P, Brubaker L, Cundiff G, Davis G, Dmochowski RR, et al. The standardization of terminology for researchers in female pelvic floor disorders. International Urogynecology Journal and Pelvic Floor Dysfunction. 2001;**12**:178-186. DOI: 10.1007/pl00004033

[20] Barber MD, Brubaker L, Nygaard I, Wheeler TL, Schaffer J, Chen Z, et al. Defining success after surgery for pelvic organ prolapse. Obstetrics and Gynecology. 2009;**114**:600-609. DOI: 10.1097/AOG.0b013e3181b2b1ae

[21] Kahn B, Varner RE, Murphy M, Sand P, Thomas S, Lipetskaia L, et al. Transvaginal mesh compared with native tissue repair for pelvic organ prolapse. Obstetrics and Gynecology. 2022;**139**:975-985. DOI: 10.1097/AOG.0000000000004794

[22] Developed by the Joint Writing Group of the American Urogynecologic Society and the International Urogynecological Association. Joint position statement on the management of mesh-related complications for the FPMRS specialist. International Urogynecology Journal. 2020;**31**:679-694. DOI: 10.1007/s00192-020-04248-x

[23] Padoa A, Braga A, Fligelman T, Athanasiou S, Phillips C, Salvatore S,

et al. European Urogynaecological Association position statement: Pelvic organ prolapse surgery. Urogynecology (Philadelphia, Pa). 2023;**29**:703-716. DOI: 10.1097/SPV.0000000000001396

[24] Boston Scientific Corporation. Uphold LTE Vaginal Support System (P180018) and Xenform Soft Tissue Reapir System (P180021). Prepared for Obstetrics and Gynecology Devices Panel of the Medical Devices Advisory Committee: Transvaginal Mesh for Anterior Prolapse Repair [Internet]. 2019. Available from: https://www.fda.gov/media/122867/download [Accessed: 10 October 2024]

[25] de Tayrac R, Sentilhes L. Complications of pelvic organ prolapse surgery and methods of prevention. International Urogynecology Journal. 2013;**24**:1859-1872. DOI: 10.1007/s00192-013-2177-9

[26] Sayer T, Lim J, Gauld JM, Hinoul P, Jones P, Franco N, et al. Medium-term clinical outcomes following surgical repair for vaginal prolapse with tension-free mesh and vaginal support device. International Urogynecology Journal. 2012;**23**:487-493. DOI: 10.1007/s00192-011-1600-3

[27] Margulies RU, Lewicky-Gaupp C, Fenner DE, McGuire EJ, Clemens JQ, Delancey JOL. Complications requiring reoperation following vaginal mesh kit procedures for prolapse. American Journal of Obstetrics and Gynecology. 2008;**199**(678):e1-e4. DOI: 10.1016/j.ajog.2008.07.049

[28] Luo DY, Yang TX, Shen H. Long term follow-up of transvaginal anatomical implant of mesh in pelvic organ prolapse. Scientific Reports. 2018;**8**:2829. DOI: 10.1038/s41598-018-21090-w

[29] Cobb WS, Burns JM, Peindl RD, Carbonell AM, Matthews BD,

Kercher KW, et al. Textile analysis of heavy weight, mid-weight, and light weight polypropylene mesh in a porcine ventral hernia model. The Journal of Surgical Research. 2006;**136**:1-7. DOI: 10.1016/j.jss.2006.05.022

[30] Baylón K, Rodríguez-Camarillo P, Elías-Zúñiga A, Díaz-Elizondo JA, Gilkerson R, Lozano K. Past, present and future of surgical meshes: A review. Membranes. 2017;**7**:47. DOI: 10.3390/membranes7030047

[31] Brown CN, Finch JG. Which mesh for hernia repair? Annals of the Royal College of Surgeons of England. 2010;**92**:272-278. DOI: 10.1308/003588410X12664192076296

[32] Bellón JM, Jurado F, García-Honduvilla N, López R, Carrera-San Martín A, Buján J. The structure of a biomaterial rather than its chemical composition modulates the repair process at the peritoneal level. American Journal of Surgery. 2002;**184**:154-159. DOI: 10.1016/s0002-9610(02)00907-8

[33] Nazemi TM, Kobashi KC. Complications of grafts used in female pelvic floor reconstruction: Mesh erosion and extrusion. Indian Journal of Urology: IJU: Journal of the Urological Society of India. 2007;**23**:153-160. DOI: 10.4103/0970-1591.32067

[34] Mangir N, Roman S, Chapple CR, MacNeil S. Complications related to use of mesh implants in surgical treatment of stress urinary incontinence and pelvic organ prolapse: Infection or inflammation? World Journal of Urology. 2020;**38**:73-80. DOI: 10.1007/s00345-019-02679-w

[35] Knight KM, Moalli PA, Abramowitch SD. Preventing mesh pore collapse by designing mesh pores with auxetic geometries: A comprehensive

evaluation via computational modeling. Journal of Biomechanical Engineering. 2018;**140**:0510051-0510058. DOI: 10.1115/1.4039058

[36] Barone WR, Moalli PA, Abramowitch SD. Textile properties of synthetic prolapse mesh in response to uniaxial loading. American Journal of Obstetrics and Gynecology. 2016;**215**(326):e1-e9. DOI: 10.1016/j. ajog.2016.03.023

[37] Food and Drug Administration. FDA Takes Action to Protect Women's Health, Orders Manufacturers of Surgical Mesh Intended for Transvaginal Repair of Pelvic Organ Prolapse to Stop Selling All Devices [Internet]. 2019. Available from: https://www.fda.gov/news-events/press-announcements/fda-takes-action-protect-womens-health-orders-manufacturers-surgical-mesh-intended-transvaginal [Accessed: 25 September 2024]

[38] Nager CW, Visco AG, Richter HE, Rardin CR, Komesu Y, Harvie HS, et al. Effect of sacrospinous hysteropexy with graft vs vaginal hysterectomy with uterosacral ligament suspension on treatment failure in women with uterovaginal prolapse: 5-year results of a randomized clinical trial. American Journal of Obstetrics and Gynecology. 2021;**225**:153.e1-153.e31. DOI: 10.1016/j. ajog.2021.03.012

[39] Cervigni M, Ercoli A, Levy G. Cadaver study of anchorless implant for the treatment of anterior and apical vaginal wall prolapse. European Journal of Obstetrics & Gynecology and Reproductive Biology. 2017;**210**:173-176. DOI: 10.1016/j.ejogrb.2016.12.031

[40] Levy G, Padoa A, Fekete Z, Bartfai G, Pajor L, Cervigni M. Self-retaining support implant: An anchorless system for the treatment of pelvic organ prolapse—2-year follow-up. International Urogynecology Journal. 2018;**29**:709-714. DOI: 10.1007/s00192-017-3415-3

[41] Levy G, Padoa A, Marcus N, Beck A, Fekete Z, Cervigni M. Anchorless implant for the treatment of advanced anterior and apical vaginal prolapse—Medium term follow up. European Journal of Obstetrics & Gynecology and Reproductive Biology. 2020;**246**:55-59. DOI: 10.1016/j.ejogrb.2020.01.005

[42] Levy G, Galin A, Padoa A, Marciano G, Marcus N, Fekete Z, et al. Surgery for pelvic organ prolapse: The case for an anchorless implant repair. International Journal of Current Medical and Pharmaceutical Research. 2019;**5**:4781-4785. DOI: 10.24327/23956429. ijcmpr201912801

[43] Levy G, Beck A, Zines Y, Shaubi-Rosen M, Shemer O, Pensky M. Non-fixative vaginal implant for repairing advanced pelvic prolapse. Harefuah. 2022;**161**:736-742

Chapter 4

Laparoscopic Techniques in the Management of Large Suprarenal Masses

Waleed Mohamed Fadlalla, Ahmed Abdelbary,
Islam Ali Soliman ElSayed and Nada Salama

Abstract

Laparoscopic adrenalectomy (LA), first described by Gagner et al. in 1992, has become the standard approach for excising benign adrenal tumours. Compared to traditional open surgery, this technique offers benefits such as reduced postoperative pain, shorter hospital stays, and quicker recovery. However, its use for large adrenal masses remains debated due to concerns regarding oncological safety, procedural complexity, and potential complications. Although laparoscopic surgery is generally preferred, certain conditions, including adrenocortical carcinoma with radiographic evidence of invasion, recurrent tumours, or severe cardiopulmonary disease, serve as contraindications. The procedure also presents challenges due to tumour size, location, and malignancy potential, which may influence recurrence and metastasis risks. Consequently, such cases should be managed by highly experienced surgeons, with the option of converting to open surgery when necessary to ensure patient safety. There is also the potential risk of injury to adjacent structures according to the site of the tumour, including kidney, liver, spleen, pancreas, inferior vena cava, and bowel. Many factors make the laparoscopic technique more challenging, including size, location, pathology of the tumour, and surgical proficiency. The major factor that keeps the laparoscopic technique still debatable is the potential of the tumour to be malignant, which is proportional to the tumour size. Many factors may result in local tumour recurrence and metastases, including risk for partial resection, tumour spillage, and capsular disruption. High-volume and experienced laparoscopic surgeons should adopt the transperitoneal laparoscopic adrenalectomy (TLA) in large suprarenal masses with consideration for conversion to open technique when necessary to achieve maximum oncological and patient safety outcomes.

Keywords: suprarenal tumours, adrenal mass, minimally invasive techniques, laparoscopic approaches, laparoscopic adrenalectomy, adrenocortical carcinoma, pheochromocytoma, intraoperative ultrasound, TNM staging

1. Introduction

1.1 Adrenal diseases associated with increased function

1.1.1 Cortex

1.1.1.1 Cushing's syndrome

Cushing syndrome results from prolonged exposure to excessive cortisol, commonly due to long-term glucocorticoid use (exogenous) or adrenal gland overproduction (endogenous) (**Table 1**) [1–7].
Signs and symptoms:
Symptoms include weight gain, skin changes, muscle weakness, and hypertension (**Table 1**) [8].
Diagnosis:
Diagnosis is made, after excluding the exogenous use of glucocorticoids, using (salivary cortisol, urine cortisol, 1 mg overnight or 2 mg 48-hour dexamethasone suppression test) [9].

1.1.1.2 Primary aldosteronism (Conn's syndrome)

Most frequently caused by aldosterone-producing adenomas or adrenal hyperplasia. However, other possible causes may include aldosterone-producing adrenal carcinoma, ectopic secretion of aldosterone either from kidneys or ovaries, or bilateral zona glomerulosa hyperplasia [10].
Signs and symptoms:
Symptoms vary but often include first-occurrence and resistant hypertension, fatigue, and electrolyte imbalances. Some patients remain asymptomatic. Hypokalaemia has been found in most cases, but recent studies have shown a less than 40% correlation. Mild hypernatraemia and hypomagnesaemia are also found in these patients. Rarely, muscle weakness and spasms occur due to the hypokalaemia of the disorder [11].

More common	Less common
Decreased libido	ECG abnormalities
Obesity/weight gain	Striea
Plethora	Oedema
Round face	Proximal muscle weakness
Menstrual changes	Osteopenia or fracture
Hirsutism	Headache
Ecchymosis	Backache
Lethargy, depression	Recurrent infections
Dorsal fat pad	Abdominal pain
Abnormal glucose tolerance	Acne
Hypertension	Female balding

Table 1.
Clinical features of Cushing's syndrome.

Diagnosis:

Hypokalaemia in a patient manifested with hypertension is the most common clue sign for diagnosing primary hyperaldosteronism. However, In up to 38% of patients, normal serum potassium may present, specifically in those patients presented with adrenal hyperplasia or familial aldosteronism [12].

Laboratory studies may show hypernatraemia, hypokalaemia, and metabolic alkalosis [13].

1.1.2 Medulla

1.1.2.1 Pheochromocytoma

The clinical manifestations of a pheochromocytoma result from excessive intermittent or continuous catecholamine secretion by the tumour. The secreted catecholamines typically are norepinephrine and epinephrine; some tumours may produce dopamine [14].

Signs and symptoms:

Classically, in patients presented with a pheochromocytoma, the triad of symptoms consists of episodic headache, tachycardia, and sweating [15]. Approximately 50% of patients have paroxysmal attacks of hypertension; however, most of the rest of patients may have primary (formerly called "essential") hypertension or even normal blood pressure [16].

Diagnosis:

Recent guidelines of the North American Neuroendocrine Tumour Society (NANETS) have recommended biochemical testing for pheochromocytoma in the following cases [17]:

- Symptomatic patients

- Patients with an adrenal incidentaloma

- Patients with a hereditary risk for developing either pheochromocytoma or paraganglioma (extra-adrenal pheochromocytoma)

The highest sensitivity [96%] for detecting a pheochromocytoma is found using plasma metanephrine testing; however, it has a lower specificity (85%) [18]. On the contrary, a 24-hour urine collection for catecholamine and metanephrine has a documented sensitivity of 87.5% and a specificity of 99.7% [19].

1.1.2.2 Neuroblastoma

Neuroblastoma (NB) is a poorly differentiated neoplasm derived from neural crest cells. It originates in the medulla of the adrenal gland and para-spinal or peri-aortic fields [20].

The symptoms of neuroblastoma largely depend on its site of origin, with approximately 65% of primary cases developing in the abdominal region—40% specifically in the adrenal gland. As a result, many affected children experience abdominal discomfort, including bloating or swelling. Neuroblastoma ranks as the third most prevalent malignancy in children under 14 years, following acute lymphoblastic leukaemia and brain or central nervous system cancers. It constitutes around 7% of all paediatric cancers but is responsible for over 10% of childhood cancer-related deaths [21–22].

1.1.3 Ganglioneuroma

Ganglioneuromas (GN) are tumours of the sympathetic nervous system originating from neural crest sympathogonia [23]. These tumours typically appear as a single, slow-growing, painless mass composed of ganglion cells, Schwann cells, and fibrous tissue. The most frequently affected regions include the posterior mediastinum (41%), retroperitoneum (37%), adrenal gland (21%), and neck (8%) [24].

1.2 Adrenal diseases associated with decreased function

Addison's disease is adrenocortical insufficiency due to dysfunction of the entire adrenal cortex, affecting glucocorticoid and mineralocorticoid function. The disease onset usually occurs when 90% or more of both adrenal cortices are dysfunctional or destroyed [25].

1.3 Adrenal diseases associated with normal function (adrenal incidentaloma)

Adrenal masses are frequently discovered incidentally and are then termed adrenal incidentalomas. Usually, the patient has no signs or symptoms of hormonal excess or obvious underlying malignancy and is usually incidentally discovered on imaging done for another unrelated cause [26].

Non-functional adrenal adenoma is the most common mass of the adrenal gland. Other pathologies may include adrenocortical carcinoma, myelolipoma, adrenal cysts or pseudocysts, adrenal haemorrhage, metastases or lymphoma [27].

1.3.1 How much does adrenal tumour size predict the likelihood of malignancy?

Research by Ross, Aron, and colleagues suggests that adrenal cortical neoplasms exceeding 6 cm in size have a malignancy rate ranging from 35–98%. Due to this elevated risk, the use of laparoscopic adrenalectomy for such tumours remains a topic of debate [28].

Since approximately 5% of incidentally detected adrenal tumours are malignant, distinguishing between benign and malignant cortical tumours before surgery is often challenging. Therefore, establishing reliable preoperative diagnostic methods for identifying malignant adrenal cortical lesions would be highly advantageous. The selection of a surgical approach is influenced by factors such as tumour size, evidence of local tissue invasion, the presence of metastases, and the surgeon's level of expertise.

Sturgeon et al. recommend a heightened suspicion for adrenocortical carcinoma when an adrenal lesion measures 8 cm or more, or when imaging suggests malignancy. In cases where dissection proves difficult due to large tumour size, adhesions, or invasive growth, surgeons should consider switching to an open or hand-assisted technique to prevent capsular rupture and tumour spillage [29, 30].

1.3.2 Impact of different laparoscopic approaches and resection of large adrenal tumours

Laparoscopic adrenalectomy, including both the transperitoneal (TLA) and retroperitoneal (RLA) approaches, has been regarded as the gold standard for the management of adrenal tumours [31]. The transperitoneal approach is favoured for its superior visibility, larger working space, and familiarity with anatomical landmarks for surgeons. Studies suggest that transperitoneal laparoscopic adrenalectomy

(TLA) is more effective than retroperitoneal laparoscopic adrenalectomy (RLA) for adrenal tumours exceeding 5 cm. However, TLA may disrupt intra-abdominal structures, increasing the risk of organ or vascular injury. Additional complications include prolonged ileus and the potential for adhesion formation. Performing TLA can be particularly challenging in patients with a history of abdominal surgery. In contrast, RLA offers a more direct approach without disturbing intra-abdominal organs. Nevertheless, its limited visibility and restricted working space can make it less suitable for larger adrenal tumours.

1.3.2.1 Anatomical consideration

The adrenal glands are retroperitoneal structures positioned at the superior medial aspect of the upper pole of each kidney. They are separated from the ribs, pleural reflection, and muscles—including the subcostal, Sacro spinalis, and latissimus dorsi—by Gerota's fascia and surrounding pararenal fat.

The right adrenal gland is situated adjacent to the bare area of the liver. Autopsy studies indicate that approximately 10% of individuals develop hepatic-adrenal fusion due to the absence of fibrous tissue between the cranial section of the right adrenal gland and the liver parenchyma. In some cases, the adrenal gland may also adhere to the kidney [32].

1.3.2.2 Anatomical relationships of the adrenal glands

1.3.2.2.1 Right adrenal gland

The peritoneal layer spanning the liver, kidney, and hepatic flexure of the colon extends over the ventrolateral portion of the right adrenal gland. The ventromedial part is located posterior to the inferior vena cava, separating the gland from the epiploic foramen anteriorly and the third section of the duodenum and pancreatic head posteriorly.

1.3.2.2.2 Left adrenal gland

The medial boundary lies next to the inferior-medial left coeliac ganglion and the left inferior phrenic and gastric arteries, which ascend along the left diaphragmatic crus. The ventral aspect is in contact with the stomach's dorsal viscera, the spleen's medial border, and the pancreatic body.

The splenic vein and artery run inferior to the left adrenal gland. Positioned anterior to the origin of the coeliac trunk, the left adrenal gland is separated from the aorta by only a few millimetres.

1.3.2.2.3 Blood supply

1.3.2.2.3.1 Arterial supply

- Superior suprarenal arteries – Originate from the inferior phrenic arteries and run superiorly and medially towards the adrenal glands.

- Middle suprarenal artery – Arises directly from the aorta.

- Inferior suprarenal arteries – Branch off from the neighbouring renal artery.

Additionally, other vessels may contribute to the adrenal gland's blood supply, including the intercostal arteries, the left ovarian artery, and the left internal spermatic arteries. The entry points of these arteries into the gland vary and do not follow a consistent anatomical pattern [33–35].

1.3.2.2.3.2 Venous drainage

In most cases, each adrenal gland is drained by a single vein. Controlling the adrenal vein during surgery is generally more straightforward on the left side, as the left adrenal vein is significantly longer than its right counterpart. Conversely, the right adrenal vein, which measures less than 1 cm in length, drains directly into the posterior inferior vena cava, increasing the risk of vascular injury and haemorrhage during surgical procedures.

The left adrenal vein typically empties into the left renal vein. However, in some instances, it may drain into the left inferior phrenic vein before reaching the left renal vein or, in rarer cases, cross over the aorta to empty directly into the inferior vena cava [34, 35].

Emerging from the hilum, the right adrenal vein enters the posterior segment of the inferior vena cava at an approximate 45° angle. Due to its short length (less than 1 cm), it is often difficult to visualise until the adrenal gland has been fully mobilised. In cases of adrenal gland enlargement or tumour presence, the origin of the right adrenal vein may be obscured. Additionally, 5–10% of right adrenal glands contain smaller accessory veins, which, in rare cases, may drain into the right hepatic or renal veins. Furthermore, small hepatic branches from the posterior liver surface can sometimes join the adrenal vein, increasing the risk of injury during adrenalectomy [34, 35].

1.3.2.2.3.3 Lymphatic drainage

The adrenal gland contains two distinct lymphatic plexuses: one situated within the medulla and the other located beneath the adrenal capsule. The majority of adrenal lymphatic drainage converges at the lateral aortic lymph nodes and the para-aortic nodes positioned near the diaphragmatic crus and the renal artery's origin. Therefore, during surgery for a suspected malignant adrenal tumour, it is essential to assess the adjacent para-aortic and para-caval lymph nodes for potential local metastases [36].

1.3.2.3 Radiological considerations

As a non-invasive imaging modality, radiology has emerged as an indispensable tool in the preoperative assessment, staging, metastatic workup, and intraoperative guidance of such tumours.

1.3.2.3.1 Preoperative assessment

The initial step in managing a large suprarenal tumour with a size threshold above 5 cm involves a thorough preoperative assessment to determine the tumour's size, location, and extent of spread. CT excels in delineating the tumour's relationship with adjacent structures, while MRI provides superior soft tissue contrast, aiding in characterising the tumour's internal architecture and vascular supply.

CT or MR angiography are necessary tools as well to visualise tumoural arterial anatomy. It is mandatory to report on variants in the arterial and venous anatomy, parasitic arterial feeders, and abnormal vascular loops, especially from the splenic artery, that can sometimes be troublesome for surgeons during laparoscopic dissection of the left adrenal gland.

1.3.2.3.2 Staging

Radiology plays a pivotal role in staging suprarenal tumours. CT and MRI are used to evaluate local tumour spread, regional lymph node involvement, and distant metastases. Functional imaging techniques, such as positron emission tomography (PET) with fluorodeoxyglucose (FDG), can be used to detect metabolically active tumours, particularly in cases of suspected malignancy.

Five common radiological signs are used for characterisation:

1. Tumour density: Greater than 10 Hounsfield units (HU) on non-contrast CT scans.

2. Contrast-enhanced CT: Evaluation includes delayed intravenous contrast washout, measured as either absolute or relative percentage washout.

3. MRI chemical shift analysis: Identifies signal intensity reduction between in-phase and out-of-phase images, assessed both qualitatively and quantitatively.

4. Fluorine-18 fludeoxyglucose (18F-FDG) PET or PET-CT: Measurement of the maximum standardised uptake value (SUVmax).

5. Adrenal-to-liver SUVmax ratio: Comparison of SUVmax in the adrenal gland relative to the liver.

Several staging systems are used to classify suprarenal tumours based on their size, local invasion, regional lymph node involvement, and distant metastases. The most commonly used staging systems include the TNM system and the American Joint Committee on Cancer (AJCC) staging system. Radiology plays a crucial role in determining the stage of a suprarenal tumour by providing information about the tumour's characteristics and extent of spread.

The TNM staging for adrenal carcinoma, particularly adrenal cortical carcinoma, is as follows based on the AJCC 8th edition:

1.3.2.3.3 T (tumour) staging

- *T1*: Tumour measuring 5 cm or less, confined within the adrenal gland.

- *T2*: Tumour exceeding 5 cm in size but remaining restricted to the adrenal gland.

- *T3*: Tumour of any dimension that extends into nearby structures, including the diaphragm, perinephric fat, or adjacent organs.

- *T4*: Tumour of any size that infiltrates the inferior vena cava or other major blood vessels.

1.3.2.3.4 N (node) staging

- *N0*: No evidence of metastasis in regional lymph nodes.

- *N1*: Presence of metastatic spread to regional lymph nodes.

1.3.2.3.5 M (metastasis) staging

- *M0*: No signs of metastatic spread to distant organs.

- *M1*: Presence of distant metastases, potentially affecting the lungs, liver, or other organs.

Stage grouping:
Based on the TNM classification, adrenal cortical carcinoma is staged as follows:

- *Stage I*: T1, N0, M0 – Tumour ≤5 cm, no regional lymph node involvement, and no distant metastasis.

- *Stage II*: T2, N0, M0 – Tumour >5 cm, without lymph node involvement or distant metastases.

- *Stage III*: T3, N0, M0 or any T, N1, M0 – Tumour invading surrounding tissues but without distant spread, or any tumour size with regional lymph node involvement.

- *Stage IV*: Any T, any N, M1 – Tumour of any size or lymph node status with confirmed distant metastasis.

1.3.2.3.6 Metastatic workup

Large suprarenal tumours can be primary or metastatic. Radiology is instrumental in identifying the primary site of origin in cases of suspected metastatic disease. CT, MRI, and PET-CT are commonly used for this purpose. These imaging modalities can help identify abnormalities in potential primary sites, such as the lungs, breasts, or kidneys.

1.3.2.3.7 Preoperative angiography and embolization

Preoperative embolization is a valuable adjunct to surgical management for patients with large suprarenal tumours, particularly those with high surgical risk due to their size, location, or underlying medical conditions. In patients with adrenocortical carcinoma, embolization can help reduce the tumour's blood supply, decrease the risk of intraoperative haemorrhage, and potentially improve surgical outcomes. For patients with pheochromocytoma, embolization can be used to control hormonal production prior to surgery, reducing the risk of intraoperative hypertensive crises. Embolization may also be considered for patients with benign pathologies such as adrenal adenomas or myelolipomas when the tumour's size or location poses a significant surgical challenge. However, the decision to perform embolization should be made on a case-by-case basis, considering the specific tumour pathology, the patient's overall health, and the potential risks and benefits of the procedure.

1.3.2.3.8 Intraoperative assessment with special considerations needed for tumours showing vascular infiltration

During surgery, real-time imaging can be used to guide the surgical approach and minimise complications. Intraoperative ultrasound (IOUS) is a valuable tool in this regard. IOUS can be used during both open and laparoscopic techniques utilising special probes. **Figure 1(A, B)**. It can be used to visualise the tumour, its relationship with adjacent structures, and any potential vascular invasion. This information can help surgeons plan their approach and avoid inadvertent damage to critical structures, excessive, unnecessary dissection, and accidental tumoural embolization, especially with lesions showing vascular invasion.

During the operative procedure, ultrasound can level the position of a thrombus in the renal, adrenal vein, and even the inferior vena cava (IVC). Additionally, it assesses the adherence to the intimal walls. This is actually very important to allow proper placement of the surgical clamps above the site of the thrombus edge **Figure 2(A–C)**.

With tumour extension in the IVC, preoperative contrast-enhanced CT studies can be biased, considering the mobile nature of tumour thrombi causing what is known as turbulence artefact. This consequently can overestimate the size and level of a thrombus, resulting in unnecessary surgical dissection.

Real-time IOUS localises the tumour vascular extension behind the liver and the relation to the hepatic veins, allowing the surgeon to place the clamp at the exact

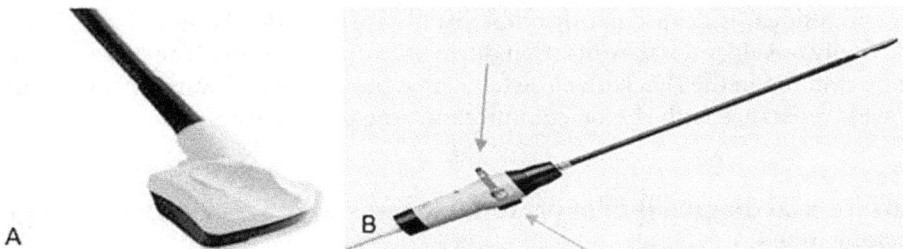

Figure 1.
(A) Surgical biplane transducer. (B) 4-way laparoscopic transduces. (With two controllers for forward and backwards and side to side motion (red arrow), with rear lock (green arrow) to keep probe position for easy use.)

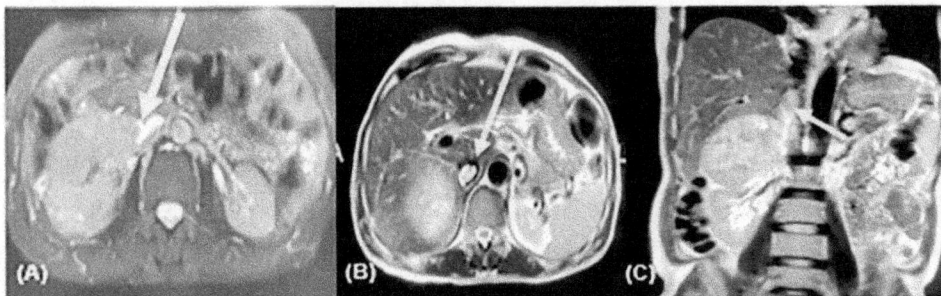

Figure 2.
Male smoker 68 years old diabetic hypertensive not controlled on anti-hypertensive medications with right suprarenal mass (A) associated with filling defect was noted in the IVC but with clear right renal vein (B) and (C).

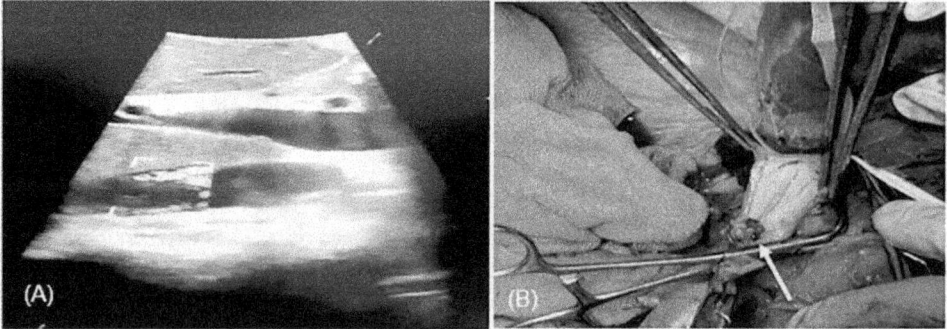

Figure 3.
(A) Intraoperative ultrasound and Doppler through IOUS using laparoscopic probe showed flow around the edge of a floating endovascular thrombus in the retro-hepatic portion of the IVC. (B) laparoscopic procedure was converted to right subcostal incision to allow proper IVC control. The opened IVC showed the edge of the thrombus bulging through suprarenal vein (yellow arrow). Specimen was pathologically proven as VMA-secreting adrenocortical carcinoma.

proper position, avoiding unnecessary hepatic mobilisation in infra hepatic IVC thrombi and avoiding the risk of massive pulmonary embolism in supra-hepatic IVC tumours (**Figure 3A, B**).

Usually, after arterial clamps are placed, endovascular tumour thrombi tend to recoil proximally due to the arrest of blood flow, allowing a safe *en bloc* dissection and removal of malignant masses.

Post resection and vascular reconstruction, IOUS and Doppler are mandatory to ensure no residual endovascular thrombi distally (prior to de-clamping) and no blood clots distally or sub-intimal infiltration during the dissected IVC. The venous flow must be restored in the IVC with close to normal pulsatility and waveform to ensure the lowest resistance to the blood column returning to the heart.

2. Differential diagnosis of suprarenal masses over 5 cm with radiological appearance

The differential diagnosis of suprarenal masses over 5 cm is broad and includes both benign and malignant conditions. The specific diagnosis depends on various factors, including the patient's clinical presentation, imaging findings, and laboratory tests.

2.1 Benign conditions

- *Adrenal cortical adenoma:*

  o *Ultrasound*: Usually appears as a well-defined, solid mass with homogeneous echogenicity.

  o *CT*: Typically appears as a well-defined, solitary mass with attenuation similar to that of the adrenal cortex.

  o *MRI*: Typically presents as a distinct, solitary mass with intermediate signal intensity on T1-weighted imaging and variable signal intensity on T2-weighted sequences.

o *PET-CT*: Typically shows no increased FDG uptake.

- *Adrenal myelolipoma*:

  o *Ultrasound*: Appears as a heterogeneous mass with both solid and cystic components.

  o *CT*: Appears as a well-defined mass with mixed attenuation, often with areas of low attenuation (fat) and high attenuation (haematopoietic elements).

  o *MRI*: Appears as a well-defined mass with high signal intensity on T1-weighted images and variable signal intensity on T2-weighted images.

  o *PET-CT*: Typically shows no increased FDG uptake.

- *Adrenal cyst*:

  o *Ultrasound*: Appears as a well-defined, anechoic mass with thin walls.

  o *CT*: Appears as a well-defined, low-attenuation mass with thin walls.

  o *MRI*: Appears as a well-defined, high signal intensity mass on T2-weighted images.

  o *PET-CT*: Typically shows no increased FDG uptake.

- *Ganglioneuroma*:

  o *Ultrasound*: Can appear as a solid or cystic mass with variable echogenicity.

  o *CT*: Can appear as a well-defined mass with variable attenuation.

  o *MRI*: Can appear as a well-defined mass with variable signal intensity on T1- and T2-weighted images.

  o *PET-CT*: Typically shows no increased FDG uptake.

- *Haemangioma*:

  o *Ultrasound*: Can appear as a well-defined, hyperechoic mass with internal vascular flow.

  o *CT*: Can appear as a well-defined, hypervascular mass with enhancement after contrast administration.

  o *MRI*: Can appear as a well-defined, hypervascular mass with increased signal intensity on T2-weighted images.

  o *PET-CT*: Typically shows no increased FDG uptake.

2.2 Malignant conditions

- *Adrenocortical carcinoma:*

  o *Ultrasound*: Can appear as a poorly defined, heterogeneous mass with irregular borders.

  o *CT*: Can appear as a large, irregular mass with heterogeneous attenuation and often with areas of necrosis or haemorrhage.

  o *MRI*: Can appear as a large, irregular mass with variable signal intensity on T1- and T2-weighted images.

  o *PET-CT*: Often shows increased FDG uptake, indicating high metabolic activity.

- *Pheochromocytoma:*

  o *Ultrasound*: Can appear as a well-defined or poorly defined mass with variable echogenicity.

  o *CT*: Can appear as a well-defined or poorly defined mass with variable attenuation, often with areas of haemorrhage or calcification.

  o *MRI*: Can appear as a well-defined or poorly defined mass with variable signal intensity on T1- and T2-weighted images.

  o *PET-CT*: Often shows increased FDG uptake, indicating high metabolic activity.

- *Neuroblastoma*:

  o *Ultrasound*: Can appear as a heterogeneous mass with irregular borders and often with calcifications.

  o *CT*: Can appear as a large, irregular mass with heterogeneous attenuation and often with areas of necrosis or haemorrhage.

  o *MRI*: Can appear as a large, irregular mass with variable signal intensity on T1- and T2-weighted images.

  o *PET-CT*: Often shows increased FDG uptake, indicating high metabolic activity.

- *Metastatic disease:*

  o *Ultrasound*: Can appear as a well-defined or poorly defined mass with variable echogenicity.

  o *CT*: Can appear as a well-defined or poorly defined mass with variable attenuation, often with areas of necrosis or haemorrhage.

o *MRI*: Can appear as a well-defined or poorly defined mass with variable signal intensity on T1- and T2-weighted images.

o *PET-CT*: Often shows increased FDG uptake, indicating high metabolic activity.

The differential diagnosis of suprarenal masses over 5 cm requires a comprehensive evaluation that incorporates imaging, laboratory tests, and clinical assessment. A multidisciplinary approach involving endocrinologists, radiologists, surgeons, and pathologists is often necessary to determine the most appropriate management plan.

3. Technical considerations regarding transperitoneal laparoscopic adrenalectomy (TLA)

Laparoscopic approaches provide better assessment for large suprarenal masses and enable the surgeon to decide which approach will be optimum for excision. Laparoscopic adrenalectomy results in reduced postoperative pain, a shorter hospital stay and recovery period, and higher patient satisfaction.

Even if the open technique is decided for resection, laparoscopic assessment will provide surgeons with the necessary steps to facilitate open resection, like release of attachments and adhesiolysis, identification of important structures, and detection of any signs of invasion. Early control of suprarenal vein could be done, especially in cases of pheochromocytoma, which decreases the load for anaesthesia during the procedure and controls the fluctuation of blood pressure caused by catecholamine release.

The transperitoneal lateral decubitus approach will offer better exposure for large adrenal masses. Adjustment of port placement is essentially to facilitate the laparoscopic procedure in large masses according to the extension of the lesion detected by imaging and after insertion of camera port.

Careful assessment of the mass and adjacent structures should be done to detect any signs of invasion of surroundings. Mobilisation of the liver is important for better assessment of the upper limit of the mass by dividing the right triangular ligament and retroperitoneal attachments. Identification of the inferior vena cava (IVC) is the key to identifying the right suprarenal vein after dissection from the adrenal tumour. Early control of the adrenal vein is important, especially in functioning tumours, and, also, helps in the separation of the mass from the IVC.

On the left side, mobilisation of the left colon and division of the splenic attachments is important for better exposure of the upper limit of the left suprarenal mass and allowing the spleen to retract medially by gravity with the tail of the pancreas and splenic vessels after medial dissection from the left suprarenal tumour. Identification of the left renal vein will be occasionally necessary before ligation and division of the left suprarenal vein.

Care should be taken during the handling of the suprarenal masses to avoid capsule disruption for oncological safety. Feedback from the anaesthesia for any fluctuation of blood pressure during tumour manipulation is very important, especially in functioning tumours.

Author details

Waleed Mohamed Fadlalla[1*], Ahmed Abdelbary[1], Islam Ali Soliman ElSayed[1] and Nada Salama[2]

1 Surgical Oncology Department, National Cancer Institute, Cairo University, Egypt

2 Radio-Diagnosis and Interventional Radiology, National Cancer Institute, Cairo University, Egypt

*Address all correspondence to: waleed.fadlalla@nci.cu.edu.eg

IntechOpen

References

[1] Gagner M, Lacroix A, Bolté E. Laparoscopic adrenalectomy in Cushing's syndrome and pheochromocytoma. The New England Journal of Medicine. 1992;**327**:1033

[2] Suzuki K, Kageyama S, Hirano Y, et al. Comparison of 3 surgical approaches to laparoscopic adrenalectomy: A nonrandomized, background matched analysis. The Journal of Urology. 2001;**166**:437-443

[3] Naya Y, Suzuki H, Komiya A, et al. Laparoscopic adrenalectomy in patients with large adrenal tumours. International Journal of Urology. 2005;**12**(2):134-139

[4] Murphy MM, Witkowski ER, Ng SC, et al. Trends in adrenalectomy: A recent national review. Surgical Endoscopy. 2010;**24**:2518-2526

[5] Li L, Yang G, Zhao L, et al. Baseline demographic and clinical characteristics of patients with adrenal incidentaloma from a single Center in China: A survey. International Journal of Endocrinology. 2017;**2017**:3093290

[6] Wu K, Liu Z, Liang J, et al. Laparoscopic versus open adrenalectomy for localized [stage 1/2] adrenocortical carcinoma: Experience at a single, high-volume center. Surgery. 2018;**164**:1325-1329

[7] Hirsch D, Shimon I, Manisterski Y, Aviran-Barak N, Amitai O, Nadler V, et al. Cushing's syndrome: Comparison between Cushing's disease and adrenal Cushing's. Endocrine. 2018;**62**(3):712-720

[8] Nieman LK. Cushing's syndrome: Update on signs, symptoms and biochemical screening. European Journal of Endocrinology. 2015;**173**(4):M33-M38

[9] Nieman LK et al. The diagnosis of Cushing's syndrome: An endocrine society clinical practice guideline. The Journal of Clinical Endocrinology & Metabolism. 2008;**93**(5):1526-1540

[10] Cobb A, Aeddula NR. Primary Hyperaldosteronism. Treasure Island (FL): StatPearls Publishing; 2019

[11] Dominguez A, Gupta S. Hyperaldosteronism. Treasure Island (FL): StatPearls Publishing; 2019

[12] Chan PL, Tan FHS. Renin dependent hypertension caused by accessory renal arteries. Clinical Hypertension. 2018;**24**:15

[13] Funder JW, Carey RM, Fardella C, Gomez-Sanchez CE, Mantero F, Stowasser M, et al. Case detection, diagnosis, and treatment of patients with primary aldosteronism: An endocrine society clinical practice guideline. The Journal of Clinical Endocrinology and Metabolism. 2008;**93**(9):3266-3281

[14] Eisenhofer G, Pacak K, Huynh TT, Qin N, Bratslavsky G, Linehan WM, et al. Catecholamine metabolomic and secretory phenotypes in phaeochromocytoma. Endocrine-Related Cancer. 2011;**18**(1):97-111

[15] Pacak K, Linehan WM, Eisenhofer G, Walther MM, Goldstein DS. Recent advances in genetics, diagnosis, localization, and treatment of pheochromocytoma. Annals of Internal Medicine. 2001;**134**(4):315-329

[16] Baguet JP, Hammer L, Mazzuco TL, Chabre O, Mallion JM, Sturm N, et al. Circumstances of discovery of phaeochromocytoma: A retrospective study of 41 consecutive patients.

European Journal of Endocrinology. 2004;**150**(5):681-686

[17] Chen H, Sippel RS, O'Dorisio MS, Vinik AI, Lloyd RV, Pacak K. The north American neuroendocrine tumour society consensus guideline for the diagnosis and management of neuroendocrine tumours: Pheochromocytoma, paraganglioma, and medullary thyroid cancer. Pancreas. 2010;**39**(6):775-783

[18] Lenders JW, Pacak K, Walther MM, Linehan WM, Mannelli M, Friberg P, et al. Biochemical diagnosis of pheochromocytoma: Which test is best? Journal of the American Medical Association. 2002;**287**(11):1427-1434

[19] de Jong WH, Eisenhofer G, Post WJ, Muskiet FA, de Vries EG, Kema IP. Dietary influences on plasma and urinary metanephrines: Implications for diagnosis of catecholamine-producing tumours. The Journal of Clinical Endocrinology and Metabolism. 2009;**94**(8):2841-2849

[20] PDQ Pediatric Treatment Editorial Board. Neuroblastoma Treatment [PDQ®]: Health Professional Version. Bethesda, MD: National Cancer Institute (US); 2023. [Internet]. Available from: https://www.cancer.gov/types/neuroblastoma/hp/neuroblastoma-treatment-pdq

[21] Board PPTE. Neuroblastoma Treatment [PDQ®]. In: PDQ Cancer Information Summaries [Internet]. US: National Cancer Institute; 2019

[22] Irwin MS, Park JR. Neuroblastoma: paradigm for precision medicine. Pediatric Clinics. 2015;**62**(1):225-256

[23] De Bernardi B, Gambini C, Haupt R, Granata C, Rizzo A, Conte M, et al. Retrospective study of childhood ganglioneuroma. Journal of Clinical Oncology. 2008;**26**(10):1710-1716

[24] Jiang Z, Zhang T, Liu X, Liang D, Zhong Y, Chan CC, et al. Multimodal imaging features of bilateral choroidal ganglioneuroma. Journal of Ophthalmology. 2020;**2020**:6231269

[25] Munir S, Quintanilla Rodriguez BS, Waseem M. Addison Disease. Treasure Island (FL): Stat Pearls; 2024

[26] Terzolo M, Bovio S, Pia A, Reimondo G, Angeli A. Management of adrenal incidentaloma. Best Practice & Research. Clinical Endocrinology & Metabolism. 2009;**23**(2):233-243

[27] Cirillo RL Jr et al. Pathology of the adrenal gland: Imaging features. AJR. American Journal of Roentgenology. 1998;**170**(2):429-435

[28] Ross NS, Aron DC. Hormonal evaluation of the patient with an incidentally discovered adrenal mass. The New England Journal of Medicine. 1990;**323**:1401-1405

[29] Young WF Jr. Management approaches to adrenal incidentalomas. A view from Rochester, Minnesota. Endocrinology and Metabolism Clinics of North America. 2000;**29**:159-185

[30] Sturgeon C et al. Risk assessment in 457 adrenal cortical carcinomas: How much does tumour size predict the likelihood of malignancy? Journal of the American College of Surgeons. 2006;**202**(3):423-430

[31] Chen W, Li F, Chen D, Zhu Y, He C, Du Y, et al. Retroperitoneal versus transperitoneal laparoscopic adrenalectomy in adrenal tumour: A meta-analysis. Surgical Laparoscopy, Endoscopy & Percutaneous Techniques. 2013;**23**(2):121-127

[32] Honma K. Adreno-hepatic fusion. An autopsy study. Zentralblatt fur Pathologie. 1991;**137**(2):117-122

[33] Zeiger MA, Thompson GB, Duh QY, Hamrahian AH, Angelos P, Elaraj D, et al. American Association of Clinical Endocrinologists and American Association of endocrine surgeons medical guidelines for the management of adrenal incidentalomas. Endocrine Practice. 2009;**15**:1-20

[34] Avisse C, Marcus C, Patey M, Ladam-Marcus V, Delattre JF, Flament JB. Surgical anatomy and embryology of the adrenal glands. Surgical Clinics of North America. 2000;**80**(1):403-415

[35] Whalen RK, Althausen AF, Daniels GH. Extra-adrenal pheochromocytoma. The Journal of Urology. 1992;**147**(1):1-10

[36] Barczyński M, Konturek A, Nowak W. Randomized clinical trial of posterior retroperitoneoscopic adrenalectomy versus lateral transperitoneal laparoscopic adrenalectomy with a 5-year follow-up. Annals of Surgery. 2014;**260**(5):740-748

Chapter 5

Male-to-Female Genital Reassignment Surgery in Gender Dysphoria: Construction of the Vagina with a Jejunal Mucosa-Muscularis Graft

Abel Mesquita, André Pinto and Marisa Domingues dos Santos

Abstract

Gender dysphoria is a clinical condition in which there is a conflict between the sex of the brain (gender) and the sex of the body. In particular, in male-to-female (M to F) transsexual patients, the cerebral sex is female, but they have male genitals and secondary sexual characteristics. The diagnostic and therapeutic approach must be judicious and carried out by a multidisciplinary team, consisting of a comprehensive rehabilitation program by Psychiatry and feminizing hormone therapy by Endocrinology. Patients who maintain intense gender dysphoria may be candidates for M-to-F genital surgery. Clinical eligibility criteria for surgery should be assessed. The surgery must be performed by a team comprising Plastic Surgery, Urology, and General Surgery. It is particularly important to build a vulva with a feminine appearance, a sensitive clitoris, and a vaginal cavity with adequate anatomical dimensions, lined with lubricated mucosa and with good patency over time, with little tendency to scar retraction. The authors present the technique of vaginal reconstruction with a jejunal graft, discussing its advantages in comparison with other available techniques and analyzing its applicability in other clinical situations of vaginal reconstruction due to agenesis, neoplasia, or trauma.

Keywords: genital reassignment surgery, vaginoplasty, vaginectomy, male-to-female surgery, gender dysphoria

1. Introduction

It is essential to remember the difference between sex, what is seen, and gender, how the patient feels. Harmony between the two is essential for human happiness [1]. The disharmony between the two causes psychological suffering (dysphoria) in transsexual patients, which may present with greater or lesser clinical intensity. Female transsexual patients have male genitals and secondary sexual characteristics but feel like women. After the careful diagnostic phase carried out by Clinical Sexology, feminizing hormone therapy guided by Endocrinologists follows. Transgender women who maintain intense dysphoria may be candidates for M-to-F genital surgery. The Plastic Surgeon may have to perform the change of the body's sex, one of the most dramatic and controversial fields of the specialty [2]. This intervention consists of the surgical conversion of male external genitalia into female ones, aiming for the most appropriate morphology possible and functional results that allow for the most normal sexual life. Of particular importance is the reconstruction of a vulva with adequate morphology, a sensitive clitoris, a functioning urethra, a vaginal cavity with normal dimensions in diameter and depth and with a lining of lubricated mucosa and good patency over the years, without a tendency to fibrous scar retractions.

2. Vaginoplasty techniques

The construction of a vagina involves the creation by blunt dissection of a cylindrical cavity approximately 14 cm deep and 3.5 cm in diameter in the space between the urethra/bladder anteriorly and the rectum posteriorly. This must be lined with autologous tissue. Several techniques are used for this purpose, each with advantages and disadvantages (**Table 1**).

The use of thick skin grafts was proposed in the past by McIndoe, producing a vagina covered by hairy skin, without natural lubrication, and with a tendency to retraction in addition to scarring in the donor area. The use of total scrotal skin grafts or scrotal skin flaps produced a vaginal cavity lined with hairy skin, with a tendency to retract, without natural lubrication, and resulted in a shortage of skin for reconstruction of the vulva. The inversion of the skin of the penis described by Burou [3] is currently widely used in several surgical centers, producing a vagina covered by skin and therefore without natural lubrication. With the aim of reconstructing a vagina with mucosa, some authors used the vaginal construction with sigmoid colon. This rather invasive technique produces an overly lubricated vagina (10 ml secretion daily), undesirable odors, and referred sensitivity to the colon. The segment of

Vaginal lining techniques			
	Penile skin inversion	**Sigmoid flap**	**Jejunal mucosa-muscularis graft**
Lining tissue	Hairy skin	Mucosa	Mucosa
Lubrication	Absent	Excessive (more than 10 ml/day)	Adequate (2–4 ml/day)
Undesirable odors	Absent	present	Absent
Vaginal contraction	Moderate	None	None
Dilatation	Required	None	None
Malignant change	May occur	May occur	Unlikely
Operation risk	Moderate	High	Moderate

Table 1.
Advantages and disadvantages of the main vaginal lining techniques.

colon that is excluded from intestinal transit may be the site of neoplasia and should therefore be inspected periodically.

In 1971 and 1972, Wilflingseder [4, 5] described the construction of the vagina with a jejunal mucosa-muscularis graft in five patients with congenital absence of the vagina (Mayer-Rokitansky-Küster-Syndrome) and studied its evolution over 2 years. In all cases, the grafts took perfectly, the length and diameter of the vagina remained constant, the jejunal mucosa remained stable, without inflammatory reaction, ulceration, or necrosis, and the secretion of these vaginas was about 2–4 ml daily, as in a normal vagina. Furthermore, Wilflingseder found that the pH of the jejunal mucosa, ranging from 6.3 to 7.6 in the small intestine, fell to about 6.1–6.7 after a few months in the transplanted mucosa and became progressively more acidic, up to 6.0, with time. It was also found that biopsies performed on the vaginal wall from the day of the operation until the 18th postoperative month revealed that the mucosa and muscular layer had changed over time, with loss of the villous structure, flattening of the epithelium, and replacement of the muscular layer by loose connective tissue, with the vaginal wall being composed of a single layer of flattened cylindrical epithelium with few crypts and a thin subepithelial layer of loose connective tissue with some scattered muscle, with a thickness of approximately 1.5–2 mm, as in a normal vaginal wall. The surface was moist and purple in color, and the wall was soft, as in a normal vagina. According to Wilflingseder, some goblet cells remain, which explains why lubrication is maintained at adequate levels over time. The harvesting technique was simple and had low morbidity, requiring only a laparotomy and a segmental enterectomy, in contrast to the larger and more complex surgery of sigmoid reconstruction associated with a mortality rate of 2%. In 1999, Décio Ferreira began regularly applying the vaginoplasty technique with jejunal graft in M-to-F genital surgery in transsexual women in Portugal [6].

3. Diagnosis of gender dysphoria

The diagnosis of M-to-F gender dysphoria must be made according to the following criteria: The patient constantly feels in a female body for a minimum period of 2 years and meets the diagnostic assumptions of the World Professional Association for Transgender Health (WPATH) Standards of Care 8. The diagnosis of gender dysphoria and its follow-up must follow the leges artis and must be multidisciplinary in nature, being carried out by a doctor with competence in Clinical Sexology, a specialist in Psychiatry, and a specialist in Endocrinology. The diagnosis must be corroborated by two distinct and independent teams. After the diagnosis is made and before starting hormone therapy, the medical team must discuss the issue of fertility preservation with the patient if the patient intends to do so. The next phase will be feminizing hormone therapy, which, due to the changes it induces, constitutes a way for the patient to gradually feel in a body with which she identifies and therefore more adapted and with a reduction in dysphoria. Despite hormonal therapy, some patients may maintain clinically significant dysphoria and may therefore wish to undergo M-to-F genital surgery and may be proposed for this in a multidisciplinary consultation.

4. Evaluation in plastic surgery consultation

Patients who meet the following criteria may be referred for evaluation in a Plastic Surgery consultation with the aim of performing genital surgery: a case adequately diagnosed with gender dysphoria; a patient of legal age and cognitively capable, with continuous hormone therapy for a minimum period of 1 year, who has a body mass index lower than or equal to 28, is a nonsmoker or has a tobacco history lower than or equal to 5 cigarettes/day, or has a history of smoking cessation in the last 3 months; is without current drug addiction; and is demonstrably already informed of the cost/benefit ratio of each medical and surgical therapeutic act. During the first consultation, it is essential to emphasize that genital surgery is irreversible. The surgeon must explain vaginoplasty with a jejunal graft to the patient. It is of particular importance to explain the need to perform a laparotomy and a segmental enterectomy. The patient should know that the surgery will last approximately 10 hours and will be performed under general anesthesia by a medical team comprising Plastic Surgery, Urology, and General Surgery specialists. The surgeon should explain that for 1 week after surgery, the patient must remain in a supine position, without raising the head of the bed, without flexing the hips or knees, catheterized and on a zero diet, with only ongoing fluid therapy. Hospitalization may last approximately 3– 4 weeks. The main complications and risks, as well as the expected morphological and functional results, should also be explained. We strongly recommend that false expectations of "perfection," functionality, and achieving full sexual pleasure be discarded. It is important to emphasize that the surgery aims above all to contribute to the patient's psychological balance. It is recommended that the patient has a period to think about and manage all the information that has been given to her, so a second consultation should be scheduled to make a surgical decision or clarify any doubts. Patients who demonstrate that they understand the procedure and the need for their peaceful cooperation with the medical team in the postoperative period are eligible for genital surgery. The patient's informed consent for surgery must be given in writing in the presence of a witness.

5. Preparation for surgery

The patient must stop hormone therapy 15 days before the intervention to prevent thromboembolism. She starts a liquid diet without fiber or dairy products 48 hours before surgery, consisting of water, tea, clear juices, and chicken soup. Admission is carried out the day before the intervention, with the administration of a cleansing enema at the end of the afternoon and another on the morning of the day of surgery. The patient must fast for 6 hours before surgery. We perform a prophylactic antibiotic therapy protocol for clean/contaminated surgery with Cefoxitin 2 g IV during anesthetic induction, with re-dosing every 2 hours.

6. Surgical technique

Surgery is performed under general anesthesia. The patient is positioned in the lithotomy position. The operating field covers the entire perineal and abdominal region up to the umbilicus to allow access to the abdominal cavity. Disinfection is carried out with povidone-iodine solution. Using a 15 scalpel blade, a skin incision is made through the median raphe of the ventral surface of the penis and scrotum from the distal end of the penis to the urogenital region. The incision is deepened with an electric scalpel. The skin flaps are fixed laterally with 2-0 silk sutures or metal staples for better exposure. The circumferential blunt dissection of the skin of the penis is performed along the plane of the superficial penile fascia.

A lateral longitudinal incision is then made in the deep penile fascia, respectively in the right and left corpus cavernosum, with circumferential blunt dissection in this plane to isolate the corpora cavernosa while preserving the neurovascular pedicle of the dorsal artery, vein, and nerve of the penis to create a neuro-sensitive flap of the glans. The distal section of the penile urethra and the corpora cavernosa is then performed: catheterization with a urinary silicone probe no. 18, dissection of the penile urethra respecting the corpus spongiosum and separating it from the corpora cavernosa, proximal dissection of the corpora cavernosa up to its origin in the crus penis with section, and its transfixive ligation with Vicryl 2-0 thread. The corpora cavernosa are then removed, and orchidectomy is performed. Hemostasis must be meticulous at each of these steps.

The cavity for the neovagina is then constructed with a scissor section of the perineal raphe limited to 1 cm between the bulbospongiosus and external anal sphincter muscles. After sectioning the perineal raphe, blunt digital dissection should continue proximally and obliquely in an anterior direction in the plane between the bladder and the rectum, creating a cavity 14 cm deep and 3.5 cm in diameter. The introduction of a vaginal speculum in the neo-cavity then allows the inspection of the area and review of the hemostasis.

The distal dissection of the neuro-sensitive flap of the glans is then completed, which is reduced by a W-V incision to create the clitoris, extending on each side by two flaps of prepuce measuring approximately 3 cm by 1 cm, which will reconstruct the internal face of the labia minora.

Access to the abdominal cavity is then performed through the superficial fascia plane of the suprapubic approach to perform segmental enterectomy. A segment of jejunum measuring approximately 15–30 cm in length is harvested (**Figure 1**) with end-to-end jejunal anastomosis and closure of the abdominal cavity. The jejunum segment is then washed abundantly with saline, with meticulous circumferential removal of the entire peritoneum (**Figure 2**), sectioned longitudinally by the edge opposite the mesentery, and

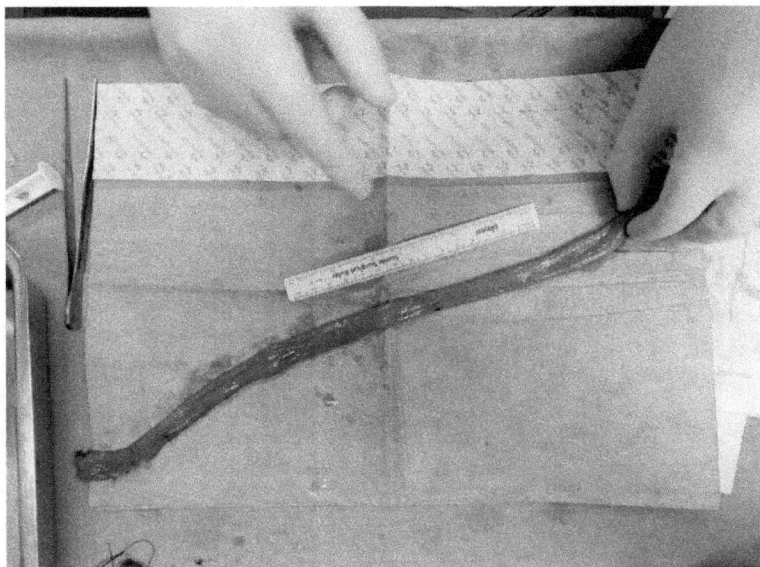

Figure 1.
Jejunum segment.

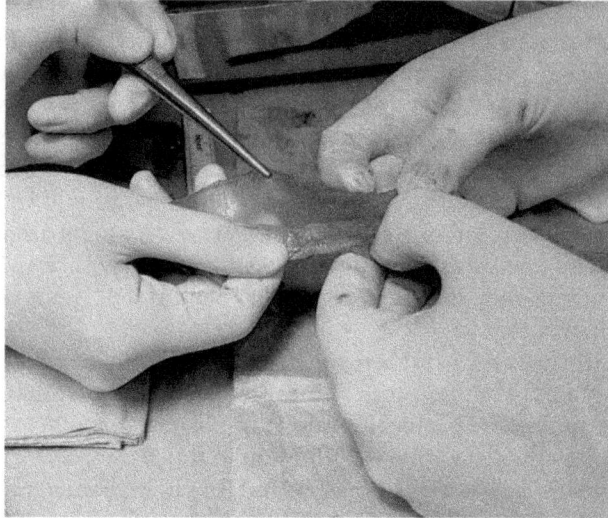

Figure 2.
Removal of the serosa (visceral peritoneum).

folded over a transparent acrylic perforated mold with continuous sutures on each side with 4-0 Vicryl thread, with the mucosal surface in contact with the mold (**Figure 3**). The authors remove the peritoneum from the jejunum starting from the mesentery line, where the cleavage plane is easily found, and then perform a 360° circumferential manual detachment according to the technique demonstrated in Video 1, https://shorturl. at/qlVMQ. It is very important to proceed with the thorough and complete removal of the peritoneum to ensure the imbibition and subsequent capillary inosculation of the graft. In the authors' experience, the small caliber of the jejunum does not constitute an anatomical limitation, since when removing the peritoneum and cutting the jejunum longitudinally along the line of the mesentery, the available tissue expands considerably.

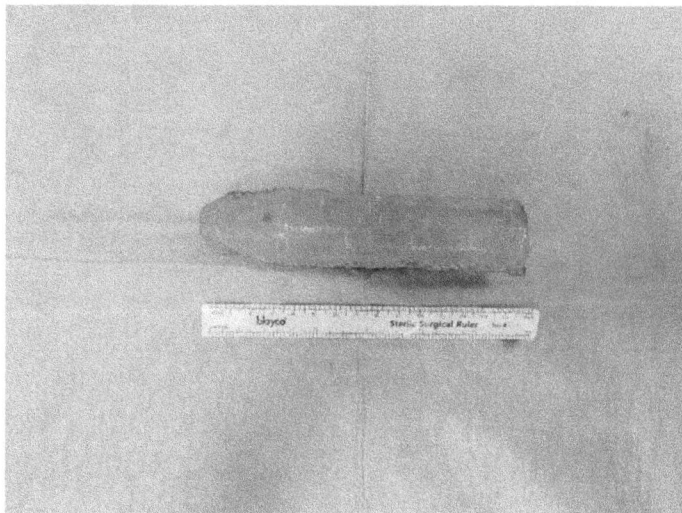

Figure 3.
Mold coating with the jejunum graft.

Furthermore, when folded transversely upon itself, it allows the entire diameter and length of the vaginal mold to be covered easily.

The jejunum-coated mold is then placed in the neovaginal cavity and fixed at the level of the introitus with 2-0 silk pull-out sutures between the mold and the muscular and cutaneous plane in order to exert moderate pressure on the mold to facilitate graft nutrition by imbibition and capillary inosculation. The penile skin flap is then advanced posteriorly to reconstruct the pubic region, external surface of the labia minora, and vaginal introitus, securing this flap with 2-0 Vicryl rapide stitches to the skin around the introitus (**Figure 4**). The anatomical location of the anterior labial commissure point is determined at the intersection of two lines drawn medially along the path of the gracilis muscles. The clitoris is positioned 3 cm posteriorly to this point, medially sectioning the penile skin flap up to this level and advancing the neuro-sensitive clitoral flap into a subdermal tunnel and fixing it with a pull-out suture using a 3-0 Vicryl rapide stitch, a maneuver that fixes and invaginates the clitoris, thus reconstructing the *praeputium* clitoridis. The preputial flaps reconstruct the inner face of the labia minora, performing a continuous suture with Vicryl rapide 4-0 to the adjacent penile skin flap. The urethra is sectioned longitudinally and posteriorly up to the level of the clitoris and spatulated, performing a continuous hemostatic suture with PDS 4-0 thread from the spongy urethra to the urethral mucosa. Using a PDS 4-0 thread, the urethral mucosa is sutured to the clitoris anteriorly, to the edge of the preputial flaps medially, and to the jejunal mucosa of the vaginal contour posteriorly. Finally, the medial face of the scrotal flaps is de-epidermized and internally submerged and fixed with non-resorbable 2-0 monofilament thread to the urogenital diaphragmatic fascia, which allows the reconstruction of the thickness of the labia majora. The cutaneous edge of the labia majora is then sutured medially to the skin flap of the outer edge of the labia minora with a continuous 3-0 Vicryl rapide suture.

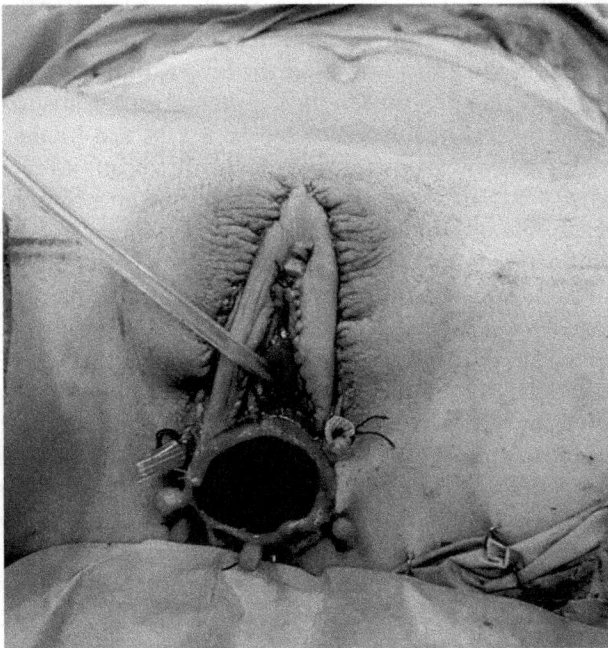

Figure 4.
Final appearance of the vulva and vagina.

Two micro-fluted drains are placed in the introitus region and properly fixed with 2-0 silk stitches. The urethral orifice is packed with greasy gauze and immobilized with a transfixive stitch between the labia minora using 2-0 silk. The surgery ends with the application of an occlusive dressing with dry compresses and fixation of the catheter with adhesive to the skin of the hypogastric region.

7. Postoperative care

After a few hours in the postoperative care unit, the patient can return to her hospital bed. For 1 week, the patient should remain in a supine position, without raising the head of the bed and without flexing the hips or knees, to avoid movements and positions that could harm the soaking and capillary inosculation of the jejunal mucosa graft or compression of the urethra by the vaginal mold that could cause necrosis of the urethra and consequent urethral fistula. We recommend prophylactic maintenance of antibiotic therapy with Cefoxitin for 7 days. We perform prophylaxis of deep vein thrombosis and pulmonary thromboembolism with intermittent pneumatic compression devices. We do not perform therapy with low molecular weight heparin due to the risk of bleeding. It is advisable to use an anti-decubitus mattress and moderate partial periodic lateralization of the patient.

We prescribe a 0 diet for the first 3 days and a liquid diet without fiber between the 4th and 7th day. The surgeon should change the dry pads inside the cast daily, which normally exhibit only moderate serous exudate that reflects the normal mucous secretion of the jejunal mucosa. Since the mold is transparent, it is possible to evaluate the color of the mucosa. Serum levels of C-reactive protein, albumin, and total proteins, as well as blood count, should be monitored every 2 days, as well as daily body temperature. In the authors' experience, moderate elevation of C-reactive protein is normal in the first postoperative week, and its normalization after the 7th day is the most reliable indicator of jejunal mucosa graft stabilization.

The authors do not fix the graft but rather the acrylic mold, which is sutured transfixively under moderate pressure to the vaginal introitus, ensuring firm contact between the graft and the bed of the neovagina cavity. On the 7th day, the mold is removed by sectioning the transfixive sutures to the introitus and facilitated by the mucous secretion itself. At this stage, the graft is attached and completely adherent to its bed, with no evidence of any prolapse. The acrylic mold is replaced by a semirigid mold wrapped in two lubricated condoms. The patient can then sit in a chair next to the bed and subsequently walk for short periods, increasing according to tolerance. The mold must remain continuously in the neovagina to maintain the patency of the cavity. The external condom must be changed whenever the mold is removed and reinserted, for example, after fecal elimination. The cleaning of the skin in the perineal region must be carefully carried out by the nursing team. The semirigid mold must be lubricated at each reintroduction with a mixture of aqueous gel + tranexamic acid + sucralfate. Tranexamic acid allows the control of small hemorrhagic foci, and sucralfate favors the healing and stabilization of the jejunal mucosa.

On the 21st day, the vaginal cavity should be inspected with a vaginal speculum to check the integrity of the mucosa and the absence of a urethral fistula. The patient starts a liquid diet with fiber on the 7th day and can walk after this phase. After the 21st day, the urinary catheter can be removed. The patient should then be instructed on how to remove and replace the vaginal mold, after which she can be discharged from the hospital.

Follow-up appointments should be scheduled according to clinical progress, every 2 weeks for the first 3 months. The semirigid mold is used permanently for the first month. In the 2nd month, the patient begins using a silicone mold measuring 14 cm long by 3.5 cm, which must be inserted lubricated with aqueous gel 3 times a day in the second month, 2 times a day in the 3rd month, and 1 time a day after the 3rd month. The patency of the neovagina must be permanently monitored by the patient, and this protocol can be adjusted according to the evolution of each case. The introduction of the silicone mold once a day should continue for life as a permanent rehabilitation program that guarantees the patency of the vaginal cavity. The patient should not have sexual intercourse in the first 6 months after surgery until the mucosa and introitus are completely stabilized.

The authors have evaluated vaginal lubrication in the postoperative period of their patients through gynecological examination with a speculum, noting the presence of a smooth, pink, and elastic mucosa coated with transparent mucus in adequate quantity at the entrance of the vulva and in the vaginal canal, which allows the lubrication of the speculum itself.

8. Results and complications

The authors have applied the jejunal graft vaginoplasty technique in their clinical practice since 2022 to the present in three clinical cases of female transsexual patients. With follow-up times of 28 months, 12 months, and 1 month postoperatively, the three patients presented good patency of the vaginal cavity, measuring 14 cm in depth and 3.5 cm in diameter, lined by a soft wall and a smooth, stable, lubricated, pinkish-colored mucosa with no hemorrhagic foci or abnormal exudates (**Figure 5**). In the authors' experience, there was no graft loss or formation of granulation tissue. The vulva had adequate morphology in all three patients (**Figure 6**), and the clitoris had adequate morphology and sensitivity. In one patient, a urethrovaginal fistula arose as a complication on the 10th day. In two patients, ileus occurred on the 12th day postoperatively, which reversed with medical therapy.

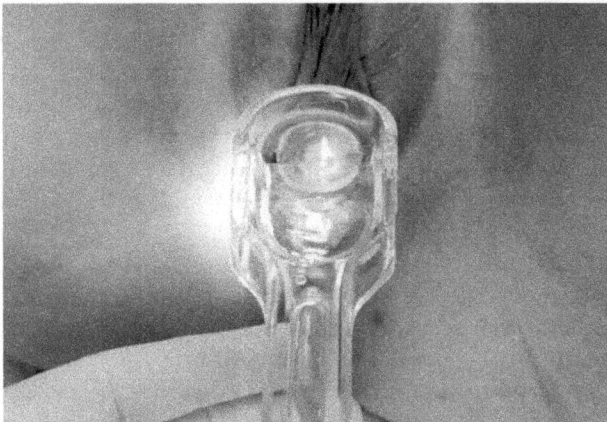

Figure 5.
Vagina with stable, lubricated, pinkish mucosa.

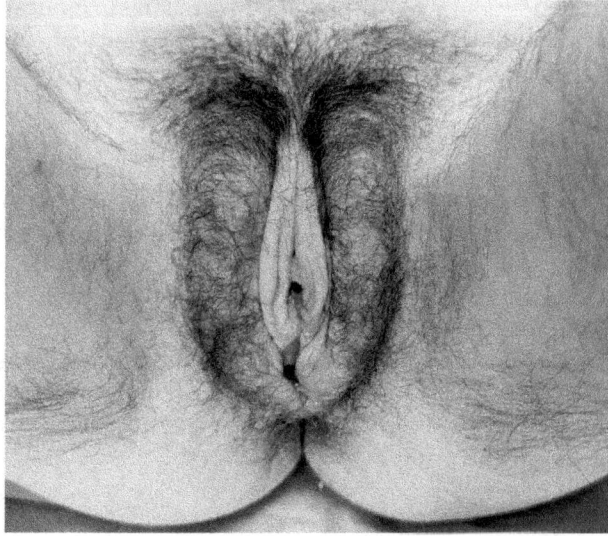

Figure 6.
Appearance of the vulva in the 8th postoperative month in one of the operated patients.

9. Discussion

The problem of vaginal construction in female transsexual patients involves not only the creation of a cavity between the bladder and the rectum of an adequate depth and diameter but also the supplementation of a stable lining that ensures the patency of the vaginal cavity. Of the various reconstructive methods described in the past, only three are currently used: penile skin inversion, sigmoid vaginal construction, and the proposed jejunum graft coating technique. The authors in their review include **Table 1** comparing the advantages and disadvantages of the main vaginal lining techniques. The jejunal epithelium regenerates completely every week and forms a stable lining that makes granulation, fibrosis, and contracture less likely to occur, with lubricated mucosa but without excessive secretion and with a low risk of malignant degeneration, which can occur when the vagina is lined by chronically irritated epidermis or mucosa, as in the case of sigmoid transposition. This explains all the advantages of the jejunum graft for the neovagina. It is a graft with a healthy mucosa and the necessary lubrication. According to Wilflingseder, in serial biopsies of the vaginal mucosa performed on the day of surgery and in the 6th, 12th, and 18th postoperative months, some goblet cells remain, which explains why lubrication is maintained at adequate levels over time. The authors have evaluated vaginal lubrication in the postoperative period of their patients through gynecological examination with a speculum, noting the presence of a smooth, pink, and elastic mucosa coated with transparent mucus in adequate quantity at the entrance of the vulva and in the vaginal canal, which allows the lubrication of the speculum itself. The quality of this neovagina depends on some technical details. We call attention to the following steps: a) the authors remove the peritoneum from the jejunum starting from the mesentery line, where the cleavage plane is easily found, and then perform a 360° circumferential manual detachment according to the technique demonstrated in Video 1, https://shorturl.at/qlVMQ. It is essential to proceed with the thorough and complete removal of the peritoneum to ensure the graft's imbibition and subsequent capillary inosculation; (b) the authors do not fix the graft but rather the acrylic mold, which is sutured transfixively under moderate pressure to the vaginal introitus, ensuring firm contact between the graft and the bed of the neovagina cavity; (c) on the 7th day, the mold is removed by cutting the transfixion stitches at the introitus. The mold detachment is facilitated by the secretion of mucus between the graft and the mold. At this stage, the graft is attached and entirely adherent to its bed, with no evidence of any prolapse. The patient can then sit in a chair beside the bed and walk for short periods, increasing according to tolerance. This technique only has a small disadvantage: the recovery times. The times mentioned are, in fact, fundamental for morphological and tissue stabilization, ensuring clinical safety. When we explain this to the patients, they understand and accept. After all, they will have a patent vagina with lubricated mucosa, with a very low risk of developing cancer (contrary to the colon flap). On the other hand, the risk of graft loss, granulation tissue formation, or neovagina prolapse is low. In the authors' experience, none of these complications were present in three cases of application of the jejunum graft technique.

10. Conclusion

Genital reassignment surgery from M to F consists of an intervention in which the morphological conversion of male genitalia into female genitalia occurs. An accurate diagnosis of gender dysphoria and the application of rigorous patient eligibility criteria for surgery are critical. The essential objectives of the intervention are the creation of a vulva with a normal morphological appearance, a sensitive clitoris, and a patent vaginal cavity lined by a stable, lubricated mucosa. We recommend lining the vaginal cavity with a jejunum graft because it is a relatively simple technique with good morphological and functional results. This technique can also be used successfully in other clinical situations in which the construction of a vagina is necessary due to neoplasia, trauma, or agenesis, such as in Mayer-Rokitansky-Küster Syndrome.

Conflict of interest

The authors declare no conflict of interest.

Author details

Abel Mesquita[1,2]*, André Pinto[3] and Marisa Domingues dos Santos[2,4,5,6,7]

1 Department of Plastic and Reconstructive Surgery, Unidade Local de Saúde de Santo António, Porto, Portugal

2 ICBAS – School of Medicine and Biomedical Sciences, University of Porto (UP), Portugal

3 Department of Urology, Unidade Local de Saúde de Santo António, Porto, Portugal

4 UMIB (Unit for Multidisciplinary Research in Biomedicine), ICBAS – School of Medicine and Biomedical Sciences, University of Porto (UP), Portugal

5 UMIB's "Oncology Research Group (MiO)", Portugal

6 Colorectal Surgery Unit, Clinic of Surgery, Centro Hospitalar Universitário de Santo António (CHUdSA), Portugal

7 Laboratory for Integrative and Translational Research in Population Health (ITR), Porto, Portugal

*Address all correspondence to: dr.abelmesquita@gmail.com

IntechOpen

References

[1] Benjamin H. Honorary Address to the Harry Benjamin International Gender Dysphoria Association Meeting. San Diego; 1976

[2] Benjamin H. The Transsexual Phenomenon. New York: Julian Press; 1966

[3] Burou G. Male to female transformation. In: Proceedings of the Second Interdisciplinary Symposium on Gender Dysphoria Syndrome. Palo Alto. Stanford University School of Medicine; 1973

[4] Wilflingseder P. Construction of the vagina by means of an intestinal mucosa-muscularis graft. Chirurgia Plastica (Berl.). 1971;**1**:15-24

[5] Wilflingseder P. Subsequent behaviour of small-bowel-composite grafts in the vagina. Chirurgia Plastica (Berl.). 1972;**1**:281-288

[6] Ferreira D. Genital M to F Surgery with Jejunum. Oslo: World Professional Association for Transgender Health (WPATH) Meeting; 2009

www.ingramcontent.com/pod-product-compliance
Lightning Source LLC
Chambersburg PA
CBHW081334190326
41458CB00018B/5994